Improving Male Sexuality, Fertility, and
Testosterone

— A Handbook Based on the Medical Literature

Dedication

To those poor men who have been damaged and don't even know it – instead they've been diagnosed as having a fluoxetine or alprazolam deficiency and are treated until they end their lives in desperation.

This book is for you, with a prayer that you are in the future treated properly and that you get happy and whole again, at least as whole as those of us who are broken can ever get.

And to my best bud, Mike, God rest your soul. Your life and dedications will not be forgotten. Thanks for being an example for those of us who are not as capable.

Dan Purser, MD

My Legal Protection

Please check out Dr. Purser's other books – get them now before you forget!

GreatMedEBooks.com

Foreword

I am a physician in Utah with a small practice that deals with hormonal issues. I take on very few new patients, if ever. My practice is actually closed to new patients but some still get through.

Well, I guess my practice also deals with more than just hormone issues; I'm part of a plastic surgery group where I deal with complex wound and healing issues. Some days I wonder if I've seen it all and then something new comes along. Most of my patients tend to be physicians.

This is the tenth book I've written on hormonal or preventive medicine issues. In the last few years I've spoken in almost every state in the USA, often to large groups of physicians who are very interest in what I know, or what I might know. I just finished a book tour of Australia. And Japan. And Singapore. Europe is coming next, or so I've been told. Recently I also spoke at Disney World, a dream come true, royal treatment and all. Maybe Euro Disney is next. My books are now being translated into other languages such as Japanese, Spanish, Mandarin, and German to name a few and are also being sold in Kindle versions.

My office hours are filled full of research for various health related companies. And I'm still involved with my research in Los Angeles and my team from USC—all the pituitary endocrinology stuff. That research is done with a former Assistant Surgeon General (who is THE smartest, most curious doctor on the planet) and other very intelligent people whom I refer to as THE Brainiacs of Pharmacology on the West Coast.

I also create health related products with THE Brainiacs who teach at USC Medical School and we sell them all over the world.

But I'll begin back where it all started—my small office practice.

Chapters

The Problem

1. Why Am I No Longer Horny? (Why Do I Have Decreased Libido?)
2. What is Low Testosterone?
3. How Does Low Testosterone Occur and Further Diagnostic Info?
4. "Man-opause" vs "Trauma-opause"
5. What Causes Low Libido?
6. Can A Vitamin Deficiency Really Cause All of This?
7. My Wife/Girl Friend is Hot—Why Aren't I Horny Any More?
8. Why Can't We Get Pregnant?
9. What is ED and Why Me?
10. Misdiagnoses Commonly Made When Low Testosterone Is Probably the Cause
11. My Wife/Girlfriend Does, Why Can't I Have Multiple Orgasms Any More?
12. How to Really Have a Blast in Bed!

The Therapy

13. I Still Want to Father Babies, What Should I Use For Therapy?
14. I Still Want to Father Babies, What Should I Avoid?
15. Why Is Human Chorionic Gonadotropin 3D for Male Infertility Issues?
16. Compounded Testosterone Creams vs Testosterone Gels
17. Plan D: Injectable Testosterone Cypionate

18. Natural Therapies That May Help Elevate Testosterone Elevate Testosterone Levels?
19. What Other Therapies Should I Consider Besides Testosterone?

Complications

20. Will Taking Testosterone Increase My PSA or Risk of Prostate Cancer?
21. Are There Other Health Reasons to Do All of This?
22. I've Had Prostate Cancer, am I Doomed?
23. I've Had Testicular Cancer, am I Doomed?
24. I've Got Migraines, Should I Take Testosterone?
25. I've had a Heart Attack, am I Doomed?
26. I've Had A Stroke, Am I Doomed?
27. I Have MS, am I Doomed?
28. I Have Male Fibromyalgia, am I Doomed?
29. My Doctor Says You're Crazy, am I Doomed?
30. Male Contraception Options That Won't Hurt Me?
31. Will HCG give me "Man Boobs"? Aaargghh! (And other potential side effects)

Ideas For Better Performance

32. Stronger and Better Natural Erection Secrets?
33. Are Male Multiple Orgasms Possible?
34. Improving Sperm Viability and Amount
35. Frequently Asked Questions (And Answers)

Guest Chapter

    36. Injectable Pre-Mix for Impotence and ED for Diabetics
          By Nayan Patel, Doctorate in Pharmacology

Appendices/Important Websites

References

Index

Chapter 1

Why Am I No Longer Horny? (Why Do I Have Decreased Libido?)

Men come in my office all the time (mainly because their wives' sent them – real men would never go to the doctor without a gun OR their wife's finger being pointed at their heads) and tell me they are tired, or even exhausted. They tell me that they're depressed and sad, and don't know why. They ask why they've gained weight and can't lose it. They mention how they're muscles are going away – shrinking -- and when they work out they just can't get them back and how they can't recover from their workouts. They also complain about how they have to take naps now just to make it through the day.

But they never tell me their libido is in decline – they say THAT's always okay (but behind or beside them their wives are shaking their heads NO!).

Then they tell me how they hurt all over. How they can't sleep well at night and how they hate the alprazolam they have to take just get to sleep at night for a few hours. They also complain how they have recently developed digestive problems and gut problems.

But they never say they have low testosterone, instead they tell me that their doctor checked it and it was "fine."

Then they tell me how their headaches have gotten worse and worse and sometimes they even get migraines. They tell me how bad the headaches are – and I admit they can be horrible. They also tell me how they now have high blood pressure problems, and how they have numbness and tingling in their fingertips. And they talk about the weird heart palpitations that worry and their high cholesterol.

They also say their wives made them come in because they used to see 50 patients in an 18 hour day and now they can barely see 25 and they're exhausted (a lot of my patients are physicians since that's who I usually speak to in educational events).

Got it? Because I do – when I take on new male patients, I hear this all the time, over and over and over. And I get it.

These are all symptoms of low libido. And low testosterone.

I am usually polite about this, and after a brief exam (guys, especially docs, are a little touchy up front when they don't know you very well – so I am very careful and discreet here), I suggest we look at some labs.

These labs need to be fasting labs, just a 12 hour fast and water is okay. Also, no nuts or peanut butter or peanut oil for three days before – nuts, especially almonds, contain ghrelin which can cause some false lab elevations thus skewing these labs (making them look better then they really are). Also, off Provigil™, Nuvigil™, and any of the new anti-depressants such as Lexapro™ or Effexor™ (for just a day or two, so they don't flip out) as these medications will also skew the results.

What labs do I want to look at in this situation?

Luteinizing Hormone (LH) – LH comes from your anterior (front) section of your pituitary and stimulates your Sertoli cells in your testicles in order for you to make testosterone. It is clearly critical and lack of this hormone is by far the #1 reason why I see hypogonadism (low testosterone) patients in my office.

Follicle Stimulating Hormone (FSH) – FSH comes from your anterior (front) section of your pituitary and stimulates your Leydig cells in your testicles in order for you to make viable sperm and spermatic fluid. It is clearly critical and lack of this hormone is by far the #1 reason why I see male infertility (low sperm count) patients in my office.

Total Testosterone –- The testosterone that is both free and bound up (usually by SHBG or sex hormone binding globulin – see below). This is not the best measurement of testosterone function BUT it is the only part of testosterone that we as physicians can really affect or change. A total testosterone range considered normal by most experts in 800-1200 ng/dl and this is what I try to help patients achieve in my office.

Free Testosterone – The testosterone that is NOT bound to sex hormone binding globulin (SHBG.). This is the testosterone you feel and that makes you have muscles and libido and drive and lowers blood pressure, etc., etc., and etc. This is the good stuff. Doctors who practice in this field all know they don't have much luck in changing this directly.

SHBG –- (Sex Hormone Binding Globulin) SHBG is a blood globulin (carrier protein) that binds up total tes and reduces free tes – NOT a good thing. The devil in every male hormone expert's day -- it is very difficult to decrease SHBG (though being younger, more slender and exercising a lot may do it), thus increasing FREE tes levels (the holy grail of testosterone therapy)

IGF-1 -- Insulin Like Growth Factor 1 - IGF-1 what we measure when we check for Human Growth Hormone (HGH) levels.

DHEA-SO4 - DHEA (DeHydroEpiAndrosterone) is a hormone produced in the adrenal glands (triangular shaped glands that sit on top of the kidneys in humans) that has literally hundreds of benefits with some being a positive impact on libido and sexuality (DHEA serves somewhat as a precursor to male and female sex hormones). The DHEA-SO4 serum test is the least expensive but also the most accurate way to check this level. Studies have shown that a normal range for a healthy adult male is 400-500 ng/dL. Above this men can break out with a (usually large) pimple (usually on the face or head) so you don't want to push it too high. DHEA can directly effect women's testosterone levels[1] [2] but recent studies (after baseball star Mark McGuire falsely claimed it to increase his testosterone levels[3]) *{I'll use "tes" short for testosterone in the rest of this manuscript -- author}* have shown that this increase in tes levels *or* muscle mass do not quickly happen in men[4] (the studies were not directly on DHEA but it's part of the same pathway), nor does it have an effect on libido[5] but does help in the prevention of cardiovascular issues[6] and I personally believe helps testosterone formation eventually when put with the right pieces of the puzzle.

TSH/FT4/FT3 -- These are the main thyroid hormones that we test with FT3 (Free T3 or L-thyronine) being the most important - FT3 is the one that impacts how we feel. Thyroid does have an effect on testosterone levels as has been shown

12

by some studies[7]. Being hypothyroid and hypogonadal can also be a wake-up sign for *some* doctors (hopefully *all* of them) to wonder if someone doesn't suffer from pituitary disease too, so it should be taken very seriously.

Cortisol –- Cortisol is another adrenal hormone but a very critical one. If you don't make enough of this (mainly due to the back portion or posterior of your pituitary being damaged) and it's too low -- you can die (that definitely effects your libido). Too high and it causes all kind of problems such as obesity, diabetes, and high blood pressure – some other things that effect your tes levels[8] and libido. But lack of cortisol is more an issue that can affect testosterone production (polyglandular auto-immune syndromes are an uncommon constellation of organ specific auto-immune diseases, characterized by the existence of two or more endocrinopathies. Polyglandular Autoimmune Type II Syndrome is also known as Schmidt's Syndrome[9]).

PSA – (Prostate Specific Antigen) PSA is a blood test used to screen men for prostate cancer (although there is currently no consensus about using this test to screen asymptomatic men for prostate cancer), to help determine the necessity for a biopsy of the prostate, to monitor the effectiveness of treatment for prostate cancer, and to detect recurrence of prostate cancer.

PSA is actually a protein the prostate creates and elutes and when under any stress or trauma it elutes more (such as with cancer or infection).

IF you tend to run high and it has not changed (and you've been thoroughly evaluated and even biopsied – ouch) then it just bears watching, but if it suddenly skyrockets? Then you may have a problem. I have seen these quite high (>8) but they are almost always due to infection, so your doctor needs to look for that first. At this time I have never had a patient I've treated develop prostate cancer – I pray that continues. And most of my patients over time have very stable PSAs *after* testosterone therapy – this is also supported in the literature[10].

Complete Blood Count (CBC) – I do a CBC on all new patients to make sure they are not anemic or do not have an infection (especially in the prostate!). This also serves as a record of where their hematocrit started and so at a future date when I re-check this I can show them they have a high hematocrit now but do NOT have polycythemia vera (it's almost always a benign erythrocytosis).

hsCRP--(highly sensitive C-Reactive Protein.) is drawn so I can check for vascular inflammation. Have a high for too many years and you will undoubtedly have a stroke or heart attack. Vascular inflammation among my male patients is almost always caused by low tes or other endocrine abnormalities (I do not live in an area where very many of my patients smoke cigarettes which can and will elevate vascular inflammation and thus hsCRP).

Complete Metabolic Panel (CMP) – (This is just me being thorough and making sure I'm not missing anything obvious.) This is a simple blood test that used to be called a "chemistry panel" -- it checks your kidney enzymes (BUN. and creatinine and gives us a GFR) and your liver (AST and ALT or liver enzymes) along with electrolytes (sodium and potassium) and other tests.

These labs should do it to start. We can get more later if we need them.

Lab Reasoning

I do most of my testing looking for WHY someone has low tes or libido issues – I always want to know root causes. I think in modern medicine, in our rush to see more patients each day (I usually only see 5-8), we physicians skip a good history and lab considerations and throw "simple treatments" at problems. Also we're trying to meet insurance requirements (impossible to do EVERY TIME ALL THE TIME) so I choose to not be involved in any insurance dealings. I want to see what's really going on when I get labs -- all based on a good history and exam. Does this man sitting here have pituitary damage (most common cause BY FAR in my experience) causing his low tes? Or does he have testicular damage as the root cause of his low tes?

It is critical to figure this simple little cause-and-effect relationship out because all proper treatment stems from this information.

Who Says a Total Testosterone Level Below 800 ng/dL is Low?

It is a widely held consensus among physicians that practice or do research in this area that 800-1200 ng/dl is a "NORMAL" Total Testosterone range for adult males.

The proper diagnosis of low testosterone (hypogonadism) must also be accompanied by symptoms – such as decrease in libido, fatigue, muscle wasting (sarcopenia), erectile dysfunction (ED), headaches, depression, etc.

In addition I have checked total testosterone levels in numerous UN-treated males in their 50s and 60s and even 70s that have been in this normal range (certainly 800-1000), though their lab report indicates (erroneously and laughably) that this level is HIGH (leading me to ask myself if I were your average physician, would I consider removing one of their testicles?).

Who Says a Total Tes Greater Than 800 ng/dl is Normal and Healthy?

Like I said in the previous section, this a number widely accepted and known by many physicians, especially among members of the anti-aging community and human testosterone researchers.

As far back as the 1970s some endocrinologists actually knew the proper optimized range of total testosterone (800-1200 ng/dl) – see the following example:

"In six normal men who received 50 mg of testosterone enanthate every seven days, the mean ($\pm$SE) serum testosterone concentration increased from 572 $\pm$ 98 ng/dl on day 0 to an average of 768 $\pm$ 87 ng/dl on days 1 to 7 ($P < 0.05$), and was maintained at an **average of 810** $\pm$ 137 ng/dl on days 50 to 56...

In six normal men who received 200 mg of testosterone enanthate every seven days, the mean serum testosterone concentration increased from 507 $\pm$ 53 ng/dl on day 0 to an average of 1199 $\pm$ 86 ng/dl ($P < 0.001$) on days 1 to 7, and was maintained at an average of 1333 $\pm$ 144 ng/dl, on days 50 to 56...

In the seven men with primary hypogonadism, who received 200 mg of testosterone enanthate every seven days, the mean serum testosterone concentration increased from 184 ± 53 ng/dl on day 0 to an average of 1033 ± 346 ng/dl ($P < 0.01$) on days 1 to 7, and was maintained at an **average of 1132** ± 260 ng/dl on days 50 to 56[11]. "

Is Total Tes <800 ng/dL Always Low?

If your Total Testosterone level is a little less than 800 ng/dl (say 600 ng/dL) but you feel fine then no worries – when you're sexually stimulated (hard to be in a doctor's office when you're about to get your blood drawn), it probably rises to well above that mark (100 or higher).

However, IF you do have the typical symptoms of low testosterone and you're close (above or about 500-600) draw the levels again OR check vitamin levels via a SpectraCell® Comprehensive Micronutrient Panel (more on this later) or look at your DHEA-SO4 levels too (see the section on DHEA.) These men are also candidates for HCG therapy but they *should have symptoms of low testosterone* before therapy is considered. If they do not have any symptoms or vitamin deficiencies or DHEA deficiencies, do not treat them.

Why Do I Care About LH Levels?

Low or non-responsive (meaning you have a low testosterone but not a really high LH level in response) indicates a central hypogonadism (also called Hypogonadotrophic Hypogonadism)– this can indicate you have a damaged pituitary.

Why Do I Care About FSH Levels?

The level of FSH is critical in men's health especially for sperm and spermatic fluid production. Ever had a dry ejaculation? Ouch! Or had to deal with a crying couple because they could not get pregnant and had tried everything? Lack of FSH means lack of sperm and if you have a lack of LH (thus a low tes level), then you probably have a lack of FSH as well (which in turn causes a lack of viable sperm production)

FSH, or follicle stimulating hormone, stimulates men's Leydig cells to help mature and sperm cells and to produce more sperm[12] and without it you can't effectively (if at all) make babies.

Why Do I Care About IGF-1 Levels?

When human growth hormone (HGH) is eluted by the anterior (front of) pituitary it is a really BIG molecule which then very quickly (in hundredths of a second) is broken down into 23 separate other hormones – all which have to do with healing of muscles, brain, nerves, tendons, joints and immune system function. Because of the mercurial nature of HGH (that means it disappears VERY quickly as it separates into all its various components) you can not easily measure HGH directly (if a doctor draws your HGH levels directly and then just sends them off to the lab you should probably realize these are not in any way valid – so don't let them do this unless the tubes are green tiger tops and frozen on dry ice before the draw and then frozen again after the draw and etc. etc. – you get the picture). Instead we've learned to measure HGH levels indirectly via one of the most stable of the 23 components of HGH call IGF-1 (insulin-like growth factor 1 if you want to say it in long hand). It is called "insulin-like" because it vaguely resembles insulin and then when the original researchers realized that it was part of the somatropin (HGH) molecule they call it a "growth factor." It's "1" because there are several other insulin-like components in addition to IGF-1 (IGF-2, IGF-3, IGFBP-3, etc.).

All this said, the real reason a more knowledgeable doctor wants to see an IGF-1 level in this situation is to see if there is any anterior pituitary damage or dysfunction as doctors like to say. We know from Italian studies (where they know a LOT more about this kind of stuff than we do – with Ferrari wrecks and Italian traffic "issues" and all) that statistically the production of HGH is affected more often than LH production if there has been damaged, so this just adds to the picture and further confirms a proper diagnosis of "central hypogonadism.."

By the way, a properly obtained IGF-1 of 250 or above is normal in most mature adults, below that it becomes a little more of a concern for an AGHD (Adult Growth Hormone Deficiency). A SEVERELY low IGF-1 is 84 ng/dL or below (so low that HGH should be started without even the need for stimulation testing[13]).

Why Do I Care About DHEA-SO4 Levels?

As I said above a proper DHEA-SO4 levels eventually impacts libido (and tes levels) and the overall health of the man.

Why Do I Care About Cortisol Levels?

You need some cortisol to survive and to make adequate testosterone.

Why Do I Care About a PSA?

Well, I sure as heck want to make sure that this man sitting here who I am about to treat does NOT have prostate cancer OR a prostatitis (inflammation of the prostate usually caused by infection). Plus, it's just a good preventative step in care.

Why Do I Care About Thyroid Levels?

Thyroid hormone levels have a big impact on androgen or gonadal hormone levels and libido in both men and women[14], and on premature and delayed ejaculation in men. Hypothyroidism or even hyperthyroidism has been associated with causing erectile dysfunction in men[15]. Normalizing or optimizing your levels (hint: FOCUS on the FT3 level and getting it up to 3.8-4.2 ng/dL[16]) is what matters the most. And if you do take oral thyroid remember to always take lots of CoQ10 as oral thyroid depletes your CoEnzyme Q10 levels.

Why Did I Draw a CBC?

A CBC is complete blood count, and I order them on new and occasionally returning patients to be thorough, and to educate. Normalizing testosterone levels can cause a benign erythrocytosis (increase in hematocrit) that is a normal and healthy response to normalizing testosterone levels in older men.

Let me repeat this – this subsequent increase in the hematocrit is NORMAL and HEALTHY. There is no rouleauxing that occurs, no increased risk of clotting, no increased risk of stroke or heart attack, and this is NOT Polycythemia Vera. I repeat – this

IS NOT POLCYTHEMIA VERA. There is however a risk that your new really healthy blood will carry oxygen to parts of your body which hasn't seen any in a while – yep, that's certainly a "problem" (just kidding – it's really a good thing). If your doctor claims this polycythemia and wants to work you up for this run the other way!

THIS NOT POLYCYTHEMIA VERA!

Okay (my CYA), there's maybe a $1/10^{th}$ of 1% chance it could be polycythemia so for those of you worry warts who don't believe me and want to experience an unnecessary bone marrow biopsy (OH, THEY'RE REAL FUN, TRUST ME! ☺), go ahead and buy into this. And sorry for making your blood really healthy too.

Why Did I Draw a hsCRP?

hsCRP (highly sensitive C-reactive protein) is a blood (serum) test that indicates vascular inflammation. You don't ever want any vascular inflammation – this will eventually lead to cardiovascular disease (to make this simple to understand – your body lays down cholesterol plaques as bandage over inflamed areas of blood vessel) which in turn leads to a heart attack or stroke (or both) or even cancer, which can in turn really hurt or make you super miserable, which in turn can lead to death.

Low testosterone causes vascular inflammation thus a higher hsCRP. I am not going to explain this again, but you don't want low tes or death, right?

Why Did I Draw a Complete Metabolic Panel (CMP)?

This test looks at simple blood chemistries like potassium and sodium levels, plus kidney and liver function tests. I usually get these just to make sure I'm not missing something obvious or easy.

If Your Doctor Will Not Order These Labs

If you can't talk a doctor in your community into ordering these labs, you can go to my website where you will find out how to get these relatively inexpensively in your community. Please note though that Direct Labs service does not and will NOT supply a diagnosis, or diagnostic code, nor treatment, or way to bill your insurance as this service is cash only (credit card or PayPal™/Google Pay™ actually). In other words only have done if you understand this information (on the other hand you may not want your insurance or IRS to know what your labs look like). (Please don't call and beg afterwards for a diagnosis.)

My website: www.danpursermd.com

More, But On My History Reasoning

Why the Headaches?

Low testosterone increases vascular inflammation (see hsCRP section above) and so can increase the rate or risk of headaches due to sensitive vessels in your head. These headaches can be bad, bad enough to become migraines (but only in men – women get migraines almost always due to low progesterone – see my book "Progesterone" on Amazon Kindle® for more info).

22

Why the Fatigue?

Low tes causes fatigue[17] (sometimes this is severe) and makes men want to nap, be grouchy, and irritable.

Why the Nerve and Sensation Problems?

Low tes causes demyelination[18] of nerves especially the peripheral nerves (to your fingertips and toes) and oddly enough the Vagal Nerve (something I learned from the team I've worked with at USC -- see Gut Problems below). Yes, and low tes is associated with multiple sclerosis[19] and yes there is demyelination there (so major experts say that all men with Multiple Sclerosis and low tes should be treated with testosterone in order to prevent relapsing remitting MS[20]).

Why the Gut Problems?

This is from the Vagal Nerve demyelination as it controls the gut motility (rolling movement of the gut as it moves food along). Vagal Nerve demyelination leads to denervation of the gut (small bowels and even the colon), leading to a brush border problem[21], which in turn leads to symptoms of food allergy and gluten intolerance and constipation or even diarrhea.

Why the Depression?

Low testosterone often causes symptoms of depression[22] and anxiety[23] in most men. This can also confusedly look like ADHD or even bipolar disorder[24]. Even though this is all over the literature most doctors don't look at the testosterone levels and instead will put patients on some pretty crazy anti-depressants or even anti-psychotics. I think this is just out of ignorance.

Why the High Blood Pressure?

Low testosterone increase vascular inflammation, which in turn causes an increase in vascular stiffness[25]. Increased vascular stiffness means an eventual decrease in pliability of the vasculature thus increasing blood pressure.

Many of my patients (most actually) are able to stop their blood pressure meds after normalizing (optimizing) their various hormone levels

Chapter 2

What is Low Testosterone?

Whether he knows it or not, when a doctor says a patient has "low testosterone" he's really talking about LOW TOTAL TESTOSTERONE.

As I said in Chapter 1, this is defined as someone (a male) with a Total Testosterone level of less than 800 ng/dL who also has SYMPTOMS of low testosterone.

For the official diagnosis of low testosterone -- you must have both –

SYMPTOMS + TOTAL TES <800 ng/dL.

Now most men will rarely admit they have symptoms of anything (such as a broken leg or missing eyeball) ESPECIALLY symptoms of low testosterone, but their wives, sisters, moms, or kids will tell you or make them tell.

So the doctor needs to listen here. And listen very carefully.

And then get the right levels. And know what they are when they have them in their hands.

What Are The Diagnosis "Levels" Doctors Use In This Case?

These are descriptive terms denoting severity of the diagnosis.

First the accepted STRICT definition of MILD HYPOGONADISM is:

TOTAL TESTOSTERONE of <400 ng/dL (<14 nmol/l[26])

The most widely accepted definition of SEVERE HYPOGONADISM is:

TOTAL TESTOSTERONE OF <288 ng/dl (<10 nmol/l[27])

These are not my numbers, but this is the widely accepted medical limits espoused by knowledgeable urologists and endocrinologists. And most of my fellow doctors don't even know it. So you may have to educate them on this little point.

MODERATE HYPOGONADISM

These are from the data we've collected and these are a little higher than the numbers noted above (the key difference is these **must** have accompanying symptoms):

361-600 ng/dl on the Total Testosterone(**must** have symptoms, too)

MILD HYPOGONADISM

601-799 ng/dl on the Total Testosterone(**must** have symptoms, too).

FEELING NORMAL

Most men feel normal and happy (again in our experience), when their levels are above 800 ng/dl and stay there. Some practitioners believe men's testosterone levels have been dropping for hundreds of years and so that men like higher levels (2,000-3,000 ng/dl) but we're not of this school (I know these doctors are out there because several of them have asked me questions regarding this concept and told me how *they* treat patients and what levels *they* expect).

" The normal range of testosterone is reported as 350-1200ng/dl. Studies in the 1940's showed the average testosterone level to be at 700 ng/dl, 300 ng/dl higher than for men today. In the past, a drop in testosterone levels to 250 ng/dl was rarely reported before men were 80 years of age. Yet today, it is not an uncommon value for middle aged men![28]"

Chapter 3

How Does Low Testosterone Occur and Further Diagnostic Info?

In almost all cases that I see (especially in ex-football players or boxers) pituitary damage is by far the NUMBER 1 CAUSE of low testosterone.

CENTRAL (PITUITARY) HYPOGONADISM

The pituitary hangs right between the eyes and about 1 ½ inch back in almost the center of the brain (not quite but classically it's been considered as being there) so when damage occurs there it's called "CENTRAL". This damage causes men to not make enough LH[29] (luteinizing hormone). This lack of LH in turn does not stimulate a man's testicles sufficiently to produce enough testosterone.

Any trauma to the pituitary (via mild to severe head blows) can damage the pituitary. Recent studies have shown us that any blow (but especially serious blows) to the head sufficient to cause loss of consciousness has a 100% chance of damaging the pituitary.

100% CHANCE OF DAMAGE!!! WOW!!!!

Now whether that damage is significant or not (it usually is) is yet to be determined and some minimal healing can occur in the first 5 years[30] (though sometimes I've seen miraculous recoveries).

Other ways you can damage it are of course – motor vehicle accidents, snorting drugs (especially vaso-constricting drugs such as cocaine), having a hemorrhaging event (blood loss from trauma or surgery), having a severe low blood pressure event (severe dehydration, etc.), a stroke, a brain or pituitary tumor, or even any brain surgery.

I can usually determine this from history and labs – and this is important as to the treatment and what else needs to be done for the patient. I have a very active preventive medicine practice and the course of treatment is determined, to a certain extent, by the cause of the hypogonadism. The reason this determination is so critical, and needs to be done accurately as possible, is because the therapies change dramatically for different causes. For example: If they have a pituitary tumor, surgery, though rare, needs to be considered and aggressive treatment afterwards needs to be planned. Also, if it's anterior pituitary dysfunction secondary to trauma, all the different affected axis need to be determined.

The best treatment option for Central Hypogonadism is always β Human Chorionic Gonadoptrop (βHCG). This is also the opinion of the FDA, so it's not just mine. βHCG is really about 80% LH and 20% FSH (and some TSH mixed in) and is usually formed in the stalk of the pituitary of both men and women, but the prescription βHCG that should be prescribed in these cases is harvested from the placenta of pregnant women (which is incredibly rich in βHCG), filtered and sterilized. It is then given as an injectable with an insulin syringe.

29

It is critical to understand that both men and women make some βHCG – this is what the NCAA® and MLB® test for – but if a player's level goes above the range considered normal then they are thought to be cheating by taking βHCG injections. If their tes is low due to trauma, athletes, I guess, must just live with the damage.

If this is for you, then you should read the very interesting and well done articles on Manny Ramirez and his use of βHCG that were discussed on ESPN®[31] and printed in the Los Angeles Times®[32] newspaper and the Wall Street Journal®[33] – check out the references.

The main benefits of βHCG are increasing testosterone naturally as possible (in essence you're giving human LH to stimulate your testicles), increasing viable sperm and spermatic fluid, and increasing libido. βHCG is the best thing going for men who need help in this area and just requires a tiny shot with an insulin needle once a day. βHCG comes in 10,000 unit bottles and I usually give any where from 300 units a day to 1,000 units (short term) to stimulate production in new patients. The biggest risk of a side effect is to become allergic to the βHCG (extremely rare) or to stimulate prostate or testicular cancer (rare too but a concern). Some doctors mistakenly tell patients βHCG can cause some pretty crazy cancers but to my knowledge and experience it just does not do that (though many cancers elute βHCG but that's where I think the confusion comes from but their ignorance still drives me crazy sometimes).

By the way, I have an 83 year old university professor who keeps his testosterone level up using just daily βHCG injections so it can work in almost all age groups.

There is an artificially created recombinant LH (rLH), which is quite effective though very expensive, but it is available (though hard to find). At USC in the research we did we used LHRH (luteinizing hormone releasing hormone) – a hypothalamic hormone (usually created in the hypothalamus under which the pituitary hangs) that stimulates increased release of LH in some men. This is an interesting treatment (not available to the public) that involves only one intravenous injection a week and works quite well in some men we tested. It's just not available as a therapy yet.

PRIMARY (TESTICULAR) HYPOGONADISM

This is where the testicles are damaged and do not produce enough testosterone and sperm and spermatic fluid (and libido).

Testicles are damaged from trauma, or from vascular disease (lack of circulation), or from vitamin deficiencies, or from other diseases. I feel it's critical to figure the exact cause out, if possible, especially in younger men who wish to have children. If this is caused by something reversible, such as a vitamin or amino acid deficiency, and NOT irreversible trauma, it would be tragic to sterilize these men further by giving them exogenous testosterone (exogenous basically means it comes from outside).

If the diagnosis is indeed from irreversible testicular trauma then the only treatment options that will work are exogenous testosterone (cream, gel or injectable testosterone

Therapy Options

First of all your doctor must prescribe these. They are highly controlled by the FDA (to prevent abuse by body builders and professional athletes) and the DEA. Follow your doctor strictly with these prescriptions and do not vary at all so he can tell if it's working or not (at least that's what I require from my patients).

Testosterone Gels

I have personally never seen one of the gels work. Never. Had hundreds of guys come in on gels but there's a reason they were coming in to see me — the stuff their doctor prescribed was just not working. This is not to say that gels don't work – they might – these patients then are probably very happy with their therapy and do not need to seek my services (I am not a primary care physician more like a secondary or tertiary care doctor, or something like that...I get confused).

The gel is also VERY expensive which is also a problem.

Compounded Testosterone Cream

I have seen some of the compounded creams work but I am really picky about what compounding pharmacies I suggest for my patients to use. The levels need to be followed pretty closely, especially early on, just to make sure the particular cream I'm using works on the patient I'm treating – they do not always work. Some guys just don't absorb it through their skin.

And side effects of the cream can be a little problematic with transference to a loved one or girl friend or spouse being the biggest concern (transference is where the man accidentally transfers some of the cream to a child or female when hugging them or coming into contact – not a good thing). Also, as with all these therapies I have to make sure there's no prostate cancer or the tes cream could feed that.

Testosterone Cypionate Injections

Testosterone cypionate injections are always effective, always work, and are cheap. They come in 10 cc bottles from the pharmacy and almost all pharmacies have them. The shots just hurt (1 cc a week in the butt or angle of the thigh with a 1" needle), have to be done often (usually weekly and sometimes more often), and when given alone will eventually kill sperm production and libido (you need more than just testosterone to build libido). I almost always suggest taking some βHCG injection 3-4 times a week to assist with libido (especially in mixed cases). (Also, there are testosterone propionate (must be compounded) and enanthate (shorter half-life of 3 days), but as they are rarely prescribed they are outside the scope of this book.)

IDIOPATHIC HYPOGONDISM

When doctors call something "idiopathic" it's really a way to say that they do not know the cause. So this is low tes of unknown cause or etiology. This is also unacceptable in my opinion – someone better be digging pretty deeply as I believe the cause can usually be pinned down.

MIXED HYPOGONADISM

This is where both the anterior pituitary is damaged and the testicles are damaged. The only treatment option here is exogenous testosterone – cream, gel or shots of testosterone cypionate.

THE DIFFERENCE IS IMPORTANT

I think I've made the point clear by now. Treatments and prognosis vary hugely according to the patient's age, severity of the problem, and the cause.

Chapter 4

"Man-opause" vs "Trauma-opause"

I do not believe in "Man-opause" (or Manopause) which indicates a pre-timed senescence of the testicles or pituitary – I think the concept is bogus and a poor excuse for inadequate examinations or history in our busy medical world of today. As I have said – I have seen too many older men with normal testosterone levels for this concept to be factual – if a man is healthy and trauma free (not very statistically likely IMHO), there is no reason why he would have a decrease in testosterone production. I do not make this carefully crafted statement lightly, it's after writing a textbook on preventive medicine and doing years of pituitary endocrinology research. Men who have been "perfectly healthy" (again just not likely) and trauma free (I have only met a few) should have no change in testosterone levels of production or libido. Why would they? These are rare humans of a superior physiology but they're out there.

I do however believe in "Trauma-opause" which is the term I coined for what I usually believe causes the Central HypogonadismI so often see (the majority of the cases I see in my office). If you make it to 64 or 78 years of age (or older) and have normal testosterone levels then you are just lucky that you've not had trauma of either your head (i.e. your pituitary) or your testicles. Also, this would indicate you have very healthy blood vessels and are fairly fit with good musculature.

I get asked about "Man-opause" all the time by well meaning doctors but I am pretty clear about what I believe. There is a lot of confusion in the medical community about this though, but more education and studies should help dispel it. I speak all over the world in an attempt to educate physicians about this and other missed diagnoses and one thing I've learned is there's a lot of work left to do.

When I talk about pituitary trauma I am being very specific about the injuries or illnesses that can cause pituitary trauma. Remember, it just hangs there between your eyes and about two inches back (not the best location, in my opinion).

Here is a list of illnesses or injuries that can cause pituitary damage (which is usually permanent):

Mild to Severe TBI (Traumatic Brain Injury)
Any blow to the head (such as by an auto airbag)
Concussive or concussion type injury (as in football)
Any hemorrhagic event (car accident or surgery that's gone wrong, etc.)
Any severe hypotensive (low blood pressure) **event** (such as dehydration)
Prolonged severe stress (the kind that drives you to your knees for weeks)
Brain tumor (of almost any sort)
Spine or brain surgery (opens the cerebrospinal fluid and lowers the intracranial pressure)(Yes, we've seen this...)
Shock event
Snorting or huffing drugs (cocaine or crystal meth especially)(Hey, cowboy, what do you think is behind that upper sinus cavity?)
Stroke
Radiation exposure (the pituitary is *really* sensitive to radiation or x-rays)
Any severe traumatic event

If any of these traumas are severe enough, and the front of your pituitary is damaged, *then* you get a problem with LH or FSH production – remember the lack of those particular pituitary hormones can effect your stimulation of your testicles. Then you might not be able to make adequate amounts of testicular sperm or testosterone or both.

Most doctors have not a clue about this connection or problem – brain trauma and what it does so little understood. If you want proof look at the New York Times® article on Lou Gehrig possibly not really having the disease of amyotrophic lateral sclerosis (also now called ALS or Lou Gehrig's Disease), but instead eventually dying from demyelination problems associated with a bean ball pitch he had received eight years prior in an exhibition game where he had a full loss of consciousness (hmmm, the Times even printed a photo of him being drug off the field unconscious after he got beaned). Any of this sound familiar?

We see it all the time.

Lack of Other Key Hormones Can Also Affect Production

Hypothyroidism Impacts Your Testes

Have cold hands or feet? Exhausted all the time? No libido, too?

Well, you might have hypothyroidism (again can be primary or pituitary causing a lack of TSH) – which can definitely affect your ability to make testosterone and sperm[34].

Thyroid and testosterone are in some ways very much interrelated and synergistic. If your thyroid is low or inadequate so might your testosterone (be low, that is).

If this is your case and you're under treatment, and so you know, we always follow free T3 levels (FT3 and try to optimize them (when possible, to around 4.0 ng/dl). We often do not focus on the TSH alone (most doctors do and we think that's inadequate).

Why? There are hundreds of good reasons why -- a FT3 of 4.0 ng/dl not only makes you feel almost normal but also dramatically reduces your risk of heart attack and stroke (maybe even causing plaque regression[35]), dramatically reduces your risk of colon cancer[36], and so can be assumed to dramatically boost your immune system functionality. On top of all this, it can lead to normal testosterone levels without any other therapy.

So make sure your thyroid (TSH, FT4, and FT3) labs are checked when you go in to have your testosterone levels checked.

Cortisol is Critical to Testosterone Production

Low cortisol levels are deadly for you and are deadly for your testicles. If low enough, this can be Addison's Disease (look it up) or certainly at least a hypocortisolism which can affect your health negatively.

This is a very complex problem (usually caused by damage to the back or posterior portion of your pituitary – "posterior pituitary dysfunction"). Statistically posterior pituitary dysfunction and hypocortisolism is less common than anterior pituitary dysfunction (low HGH and pituitary hypogonadism or even central hypothyroidism), so it needs to be handled adroitly by someone with experience. (My observation of doctors who are really skilled at treating this is they kind of throw the book out and treat the patient's symptoms and not levels, but that's for your local expert to decide.)

Chapter 5

What Causes Low Libido?

In men low testosterone is the most common influencer of low libido but there's a lot more involved in this problem than just low testosterone levels. It's critical for men to understand this as most think if they elevate their testosterone levels back to "normal" range then everything gets good again and they'll feel normal.

This is just not the way this hugely complex interaction occurs.

Testosterone and/or libido do not function alone in a vacuum, they need some almost ideal supporting cast members to achieve good libido driving all of the interaction followed by a fulfilling orgasm with healthy sperm (if pregnancy is your goal).

Libido is an interaction of many things, mainly led by visual and possibly scent or pheromone cues (wife, who smells really good, slides into the bedroom dressed in something cute and suggestive of a desire for intimacy), which then causes the initiation of thoughts ("hmmm, what does she want? Oh, she wants to get together!"), which then leads to a hypothalamic response (the pituitary hangs down from the hypothalamus), which causes the pituitary to surge out luteinizing hormone (LH) and follicle stimulating hormones (FSH) (though for most men it's actually started surging the day of, or hours before, in the hope of interaction), then the testicles become involved and testosterone and spermatic fluid are created in huge surges (hopefully), then things happen in a controlled volcanic explosion via an orgasm (hopefully, again).

But (sorry to kill the mood here) you need to imagine the billions of enzymatic and vitamin and amino acid interactions that occur to get a man to have a healthy libido or especially to get a man to orgasm. And in any one of those steps, if there's something off or missing the whole process can stop (though I believe the human body, which is truly amazing, has some "work-arounds"), and libido and intercourse failure ensues.

This book is really about making sure all these steps are optimized in the best possible way. But truthfully modern science, and thus medicine, is very limited – notice where I said "billions" of interactions in the previous paragraph and as you'll see, we only know how to affect maybe a few dozen of these steps.

And one thing I've learned over the years of practicing medicine – it's easy through trauma or poor care of the body to bollux things up in the worst possible way. Hopefully I can undo some of the problems and get you back on course.

Chapter 6

Can A Vitamin Deficiency Really Cause All of This?

A vitamin or mineral deficiency or (especially) an amino acid deficiency can of course impact on your bodies' incredibly complex ability to manufacture testosterone molecules and sperm!

Come on, people! Creating sperm or tes is far more complex than making computers and just think how one component missing (say copper for the mother board, or silver, or some memory component) can cause failure or complete stoppage of the manufacturing process. No more computers!

Well, guess what? Don't have enough zincor L-arginine or CoEnzyme Q10 and the testosterone and sperm manufacturing process stops, too.

So what's important here? The list is long but let's look at the few we know whose participation is critical in the process:

THE LIST

Fish Oil/Olive Oil – These comprise "Oleic Acids" (also comprise   eicosapentaenoic acid (EPA),   and docosahexaenoic acid (DHA-- very   important   cellular components in the human body (actually in every mammalian body).

As part of my preventive medicine practice I also prescribe adequate fish oil as it impacts mood and depression and even possibly libido[37]. Studies have shown[38] that 2,500 mg to 3,400 mg/day of combined EPA and DHA in the oil is what is required to reduce risks from cardiovascular disease (so look on the back of the bottle top determine).

Dehydroepiandrosterone (DHEA): This adrenal hormone is also called androstenolone or prasterone (INN), as well as 3β-hydroxyandrost-5-en-17-one or 5-androsten-3β-ol-17-one, is an important endogenous steroid hormone. It is also the most abundant circulating steroid in humans, where it is produced in the adrenal glands, the gonads, and the brain, where it functions predominantly as a metabolic intermediate in the biosynthesis of many androgen and estrogen sex steroids.[39] [40]

DHEA is considered a master hormone that has been shown to help with libido, but the data seems mixed and confusing as to if it helps with *directly* with testosterone production. I believe indirectly it does aid in production and has such an impact on health that it's worth maintaining a healthy level (400 -500 ng/dl) in men.

Pregnenolone –- Pregnenolone is THE master hormone from which you make androgens (i.e. testosterone[41]). You absolutely must have it. A normal blood level is near 200 ng/dl. Usually I will prescribe 100 mg of quality compounded pregnenolone to help in this area.

CoEnzyme Q10 (CoQ10) – CoQ10 is incredibly critical to sperm[42] and testosterone production, and to such an extent that taking it should never be overlooked when you're infertile or treating infertile patients.

CoQ10 also helps in libido in infertile men[43]. Plus it's good for your heart and for counteracting fatigue!

I usually advise 200 mg a day of highly absorbable CoQ10 in the form of ubiquinol. I love NuSkin's NanoCoQ10™ or the easily absorbed ubiquinol in Qunol™ (available at Wal-Mart™ or Costco™) or Med Quest™ (in Utah at www.mqrx.com) who has the very effective original all natural Japanese CoQ10 (with which all the original studies were performed). Also, if you take thyroid (or know anyone who does) they should be on at least 200 mg of ubiquinol each day – look at Stephen Sinatra's (a cardiologist in Boston who is the foremost spokesman in the world for using CoQ10) website for more information (www.drsinatra.com) and where he also carries several different very high quality CoQ10's (such as his excellent OmegaQ Plus™).

Vitamin D3 (Cholecalciferol) – Cholecalciferol (D3 or commonly just called Vitamin D) is important in the manufacture of sperm and testosterone as has been shown in a number of studies[44]. I usually advise 5,000 to 8,000 units a day of the liquid gel cap D3. (But be aware, though very difficult to do, you can become toxic on this vitamin, so get levels checked occasionally (I like to see them up around 90ng/ml).)

Glutathione – Glutathione helps in testosterone production[45] and is probably critical in the process. Higher glutathione levels are also preventative for Benign Prostatic Hypertrophy (BPH or enlarged prostate)[46]. To my knowledge there is only one real bioavailable glutathione on the market and it's my team's RealGSH™ – go to www.realgsh.com to try some. If you're deficient and use some, you tend to feel it within minutes (like severe Vitamin C deficient patients will).

NAC (N-Acetyl Cysteine) — NAC (Cysteine) is helpful in spermatogenesis[47] – if you have azoospermia, you should be on it. It's also key to the production of your own natural glutathione (if you still have or have the intracellular equipment).

Anti-oxidants (Vitamins A, C, D, E, K2 etc.) – Again, critical to protection of the testes and to sperm and testosterone production[48].

L-Arginine (or just Arginine) – L-arginine is critical to testosterone and sperm production[49] and should be part of your daily regimen if you're concerned about either.

L-Carnitine (or just Carnitine) – L-Carnitine helps with spermatogenesis and protects the testicles and seminiferous tubules[50]. It should be part of your daily intake.

L-Ornithine (or just Ornithine) – "L-ornithine is a non-essential amino acid produced by the body. It's similar to and can be changed to L-arginine in the body. Because L-ornithine is naturally produced, a deficiency is rare. It can be found in protein sources such as fish, meat, eggs and dairy. L-ornithine boosts production of HGH, the human growth hormone. It also supports a normal functioning immune system and liver health. The amino acid works in the urea cycle, assisting with ammonia detoxification, and aids in rejuvenating the liver. L-ornithine and L-arginine support the production of nitric oxide, which is important to the vascular system.[51]"

Zinc – You need zinc to make both sperm and especially testosterone[52].

Selenium – Selenium helps with spermatogenesis and testosterone production[53].

Other Amino Acid deficiencies – there are 43 amino acids and no way to test of intracellular levels of each (Spectracell™, in their comprehensive test, looks at seven, I believe, but not the full 43), and a deficiency of any one of these could probably cause testosterone or sperm production. There are only a few "complete" amino acid supplements out there, and though I'm not a distributor of this product, one which I've had good results with is called Laminine™ (contact Mindi, the receptionist at my office if you wish more info @ mindi@aespmi.com – she's a distributor).

Can A Vitamin Deficiency Really Cause A Decrease in Libido?

Yes, many different vitamin deficiencies can affect overall health and stamina and cause fatigue and a disinterest in intercourse/sex. A vitamin deficiency can also directly impede the bodies manufacture of testosterone or viable sperm – this isn't a magic process where testosterone just appears out of thin air, it has to be slowly formed in the testicles by the Leydig cells in a step-by-step process (note that some testosterone is made in the adrenal glands but not very much). Any missing substrates or vitamins or amino acids (each step involves some reaction, or enzyme, or vitamin, or amino acid) can halt this process dead in its tracts, or at least until that substance is finally supplied.

How to Properly Test for a Vitamin Deficiency?

You can just guess on this and spend a fortune in the process while you take everything on the shelf or spend a fortune getting fairly inaccurate serum levels that don't really tell you that much (compared to the technology I am about to mention), or you can get really accurate intracellular levels that detail all the information you need.

I'd spend the money on the intracellular levels myself (and that's what I do).

Okay, here's what I've been mentioning throughout this book -- there's a quiet little lab in Texas called SpectraCell™ that has an amazing proprietary and patented technology (FDA and HHS approved, too!) that in essence allows them to determine intracellular vitamin levels. Now to be clear—I am not an owner, receive no remuneration from these guys nor am I even a spokesman as I write these words – this test just rocks!

SpectraCell™ offers an incredible comprehensive panel that looks at 39 different vitamins and minerals on an intracellular basis. This ability is mind-blowing and really can get to a number of simple root causes for hypogonadism or depression.

Their website: **www.spectracell.com**

SpectraCell® Comprehensive Micronutrient Analysis Panel will test the following intracellular vitamin levels:

B Complex Vitamins
Vitamin B1 (Thiamin)
Vitamin B2 (Riboflavin)
Vitamin B3 (Niacinamide)
Vitamin B6 (Pyridoxine)
Vitamin B12 (Cobalamin)

Amino Acids
Serine
Glutamine
Asparagine

Metabolites
Choline
Inositol
Carnitine

Fatty Acids
Oleic Acid

Other Vitamins
Vitamin D3 (Cholecalciferol)
Vitamin A (Retinol)
Vitamin K2
Minerals
Calcium
Zinc

Copper

Magnesium

Carbohydrate Metabolism
Glucose-Insulin Interaction
Fructose Sensitivity
Chromium

Antioxidants
Glutathione
Cysteine
Coenzyme Q10
Vitamin E (α-tocopherol)
Alpha Lipoic Acid (ALA)
Vitamin C

Spectrox™
Total Antioxidant Function

Here's an example about how awesome this test can be -- I had a young lady (34 years old) from California referred by her doctor for unexplained tooth loss, bleeding gums, sores in her mouth, fatigue, swollen joints, and hair loss. She'd spent (or her insurance company had) $15,000 on oral surgery consults and procedures, endodontist consults and testing, rheumatology consults and testing, infectious disease consults and testing, orthopedic surgery evaluations and so forth. I looked through her labs and consult notes (which were all very good), and thought they'd pretty much ordered everything under the sun, except for an intracellular vitamin panel. I drew a SpectraCell® Comprehensive Panel on her and found out she had scurvy (a

Vitamin C deficiency – which indeed fit all her signs and symptoms). Yes, scurvy!!! It's not a disease we see much of any more but now I've diagnosed two other cases, so it's out there.

Or the new onset Type 2 Diabetics who show up at my office and have a chromium deficiency. Hello! Chromium piccolinate is at the heart of the insulin receptor on all of our cell surfaces and if you have a deficiency in chromium those receptors cannot handle insulin properly. So the sugar cannot get into the cell. Your doctor might even say you have insulin "resistance" (actually meaning insulin receptor dysfunction) when in reality you have a chromium deficiency causing it!

Thank you to SpectraCell® for occasionally making me look like a genius!

And if you want to be on top of your game in the bed room make sure you get a SpectraCell® once a year to really fine tune your male and cardiovascular physiology.

(P.S. I've never had anyone test perfect the first time I've gotten a Micronutrient Analysis™ Panel on them.)

Chapter 7

My Wife/Girl Friend is Hot—Why Aren't I Horny Any More?

Really? You're asking that at this point in this book?

You most likely have a decrease in your libido, duh!

Visual cortex stimulation helps (yes, men are very visual creatures thus the popularity of strip bars and pornography) but not if your libido is really beat down – add the depression and fatigue and muscle soreness you have when your testosterone level is low, and you get just about no physical response even with maximum stimulation from a loving (or not so loving at times) companion.

Think about it.

The pituitary is thought by many people of other religions in the world to be a major part of the sixth chakra (psychic intuitive center) or third eye and emotions. That says it all, doesn't it? And if your pituitary is damaged, you cannot surge out LH and FSH and so will not make testosterone or sperm or spermatic fluid (all the fun stuff for guys).

Sorry, but, if your pituitary is severely damaged, nothing's going to happen of any consequence. But it's not because you're getting older – age has nothing to do with it – this lack of libido is due to damage somewhere.

In essence, you can't get blood from a turnip.

Chapter 8

Why Can't We Get Pregnant?

Usually the women get the blame for infertility, and I'm not sure why. Men also should be suspect, and maybe more often than the women – they need to have their testosterone levels checked and their viable sperm count evaluated.

Low LH causes low testosterone.

Low FSH causes low viable sperm production.

Certain vitamin or amino acid deficiencies can also definitely impact your ability to make viable sperm.

There are just a huge number of potential variables that need to be normal before live sperm appear. IMHO, it's truly amazing that we have, as a race, continued to multiply.

The Best Patient for βHCG

If you are suffering from low testosterone (hypogonadism), and you're sure it's central (pituitary), and you wish to improve your chances of fathering a child, this is the time and the place for βHCG (Beta Human Chorionic Gonadotropin). The FDA has actually approved it for this therapy (look under Pregnyl™ or Novarel™ in the Physician's Desk Reference®**Error! Bookmark not defined.,** or PDR).

It can be given as compounded (meaning made by a compounding pharmacy) sublingual drop -- which does occasionally work as a therapy for milder cases of central hypogonadism. But ideally it needs to be given as a subcutaneous shot (a tiny little shot in the tummy, or thigh, or buttock, or deltoid, with an insulin needle). I usually start most patients on 500 units of βHCG each morning, given subcutaneously. If they do not have much of a response after 3 months (BE PATIENT!!!), then I do a SpectraCell™ and increase their dose of HCG (usually to 1,000 units a day, but you can go as high as 2,000 units a day). (You physicians who read this – LISTEN – you are trying to stimulate their testicles into high action here, so don't be dainty with the dosing.) But do be patient and give the testicles time to respond (at least three months or more, but I have seen it happen sooner).

Chapter 9

What is ED and Why Me?

"ED" is the acronym for Erectile Dysfunction, which to many doctors means a lot of different things – but to most doctors in general it means "male sexual dysfunction." Technically ED means that you have trouble getting and maintaining an erection but again doctors in general think it means sexual dysfunction and don't go much beyond there.

So you're a man who's not doing very well and you tell your doctor you have sexual problems?

What usually happens next?

Knee jerk reaction is most doctors will offer you Viagra™ or Cialis™. (Notice that I did not say doctors check your testosterone or LH or FSH levels, but that the first thing they do is to start you on Viagra™.)

Why?

Because this approach is quick and easy and gets you out of their crowded overbooked office.

It's also incorrect and is very ignorant (again IMHO). They should at the least check your free and total testosterone and LH/FSH levels. That's not just my advice – it's the FDA's and Viagra's advice (read the Physician's Desk Reference® if in doubt). I believe this occurs because most doctors have NO idea what's an appropriate level of testosterone for a man.

First You Should Optimize Your Testosterone Levels

Most of the respected medical experts in this area of practice (I believe) think you should "normalize" [I say optimize] your tes levels (serum Total Testosterone of 800-1200 ng/dl) in the best and most appropriate way for you first (if you want to have more kids do this via HCG injections, or if not – via a quality compounded tes cream or testosterone cypionate injections).

Next Optimize Everything Else

Thyroid – This needs to be followed correctly by physicians. In our office and in my training and research we *always* follow the Free T3 (FT3) level when we adjust thyroid levels. If it's safe cardiovascularly, one should always try to elevate FT3 level to optimal levels (3.8-4.2 ng/dl). Why not? If a patient has to take thyroid, you might as well make sure they take *enough*, right?

At a FT3 of approximately 4.0, a number of really good things can happen:

1. Plaque regression occurs from arteries (coronary, carotid, and penile, too)[54].
2. You get a big decrease in breast[55] AND lung cancer[56].
3. It's easier to, and you'll have more energy to, exercise and/or have sex or intercourse.
4. Your cholesterol and triglycerides will drop to normal (thus the plaque regression in #1).
5. This can really help with testosterone and sperm production[57] -- sometimes making it normal!

Remember and WARNING – you must take lots of CoQ10 when you take oral thyroid or you will deplete your CoQ10 levels. I see lots of patients who are taking thyroid yet are exhausted all the time. When you start them on a good quality CoQ10 (like Qunol™ – I will have them take 4 or 5 a day the first week, then 2 a day thereafter), 95% of the time they feel dramatically better with more energy and endurance and stamina. Go to Stephen Sinatra MD's website for more information – he's a cardiologist in Boston who is considered by many to be the top expert in the USA on CoQ10 use.

Simvastatin – What an odd choice right? Hear me out. Statins are not the most popular things out there (because of the muscle aches or myopathy that can and often does occur) but if you're going to take one, the only one to take (in my opinion) is simvastatin. Simvastatin is both the most natural statin out there and the most lipophilic[58] and is incredibly cheap. Simvastatin also clearly causes some of the best plaque regression out there[59]. I usually prescribe 80 mg a day (the maximum dose) right out of the gate (why not? Just go for it! Don't namby pamby it up), but make patients swear that they will take at least 2 Qunols® (or their equivalent) a day while they're on it AND we check LFTs (liver function tests) every 3 months – I also usually don't prescribe it for longer then 9 months at a time.

Why the Qunol™? For the myalgias and the myopathy – we believe it's due to the statin using up the CoQ10 in the mitochondria, this then causes the muscles to become inflamed and hurt. I have never seen myalgia or myopathy when the simvastatin is taken with adequate CoQ10.

Fish Oil -- make sure you're on adequate DHA and EPA dosages (2,500 mg a day as a total of the two is the *minimum* dose of EPA and DHA per day, 5,000 if you have known cardiovascular disease). My favorite fish oil currently is Arctic Pure™ Source Naturals™ Omega-3 Ultra Potency Fish Oil™ available at www.vitacost.com. The truth is research says oleic acid/DHA/EPA (all fish oil components) does NOT help build spermatic fluid or testosterone[60], but they DO help prevent you from having a heart attack or stroke (major bummer while you're having sex with the missus).

Vitamins -- get a SpectraCell® to determine what amino acids, vitamins, and minerals you need. It's really critical at this point to make sure you're taking adequate L-arginine and other amino acids (currently I like Pro-Argi-9™ and/or Arginine-Plus™ – a scoop a day).

Chapter 10

Misdiagnoses Commonly Made When Low Testosterone Is Probably the Cause

I wish that more physicians would do a more thorough evaluation before giving someone a diagnosis that will make them pretty much uninsurable for the rest of their life (plus probably unemployable and probably unmarriageable, too) and pretty untreatable. The following are misdiagnoses I often deal with when instead these young men have low testosterone (usually severely low) and have had some hard trauma (car wreck, football concussion, etc.) to which we can trace it back:

Bipolar Disorder

Really? How can a 23 or 34 year old all of a sudden be given the *new* diagnosis of "bipolar disorder," when technically the diagnosis requires the *first* episode or break to occur prior to age 15?

And inevitably the medications (lithium, valproate, carbamazepine, gabapentin, etc.) used to treat this condition fail miserably and make these patients miserable, too. If you've been given this diagnosis (you're a patient) or have been *giving* out this diagnosis (you're a doctor), then for heaven's sakes check testosterone levels (low levels of free tes have been associated with bipolar symptoms[61] – plus I see this often) – see what's happening down there!

Depression or even Major Depression

I believe men's testosterone levels should always be checked prior to initiating anti-depressant therapy? Why? Why not? It's such a common and relatively easily treatable cause of depression[62] that benefits the man in so many ways *other* than mood, and it's often the appropriate thing to do. BUT most doctors are rushed nowadays and so they just throw some fluoxetine at the problem and think that's good. We, on the other hand, always try to go a little deeper and take a really good history and ask a lot of questions (we usually take at least an hour or more to dig in there and figure things out). This really helps because most men are a little reluctant to admit their libido is suffering.

Before the advent of Prozac™ in the early 80's (after which any family physician or GP could easily and quickly prescribe) most psychiatrists were very careful and thorough and would look at a number of hormone issues (remember who first initiated Cytomel™ therapy?) prior to starting patients on the harsh anti-depressants that were then used (and are often used today).

Now they seem to be quick to jump to conclusions such as that patients are "magically" and suddenly depressed (ignoring that head trauma they had in that car wreck three months before)(or they call it a post-concussion syndrome – which we feel is more accurately called PITUITARY DAMAGE), and then start them on the newer antidepressants (which we believe may make the situation worse by what effect they have on the already damaged pituitary).

We see men with low testosterone get very happy when they get normalized levels – most (after a few months and under doctors supervision) end up stopping their anti-depressants.

As a matter of fact I think I have only a couple of patients who take anti-depressants after nine months or so in our office (okay, I must be doing something wrong with those patients).

ADHD (Attention Deficit Hyperactivity Disorder)

I think most cases of adult ADHD (but not with childhood ADHD since I have no experience in that area) or at least all the ones I've ever seen, have acutely low testosterone levels (usually from some relatively recent traumas).

Hmmmm, if you wish to see a guy get *really* focused (I call this the "hunter gatherer response") then increase their testosterone levels to high normal – they usually become *very* focused and intent on finding a wife, or significant other, or girlfriend, or whatever, but boy are they suddenly very focused.

No ADHD there, nope, none at all.

Studies have shown that men who have high testosterone levels versus those with no testosterone, make much quicker and more accurate decisions[63]. Guys with low testosterone become apathetic and lack responsiveness. Guys with excellent testosterone levels tend to be very focused, and intent – decision-making speed and skill matter here as they hunt, or go to war, or to bed.

And so do optimal testosterone levels.

Chapter 11

My Wife/Girlfriend Does, Why Can't I Have Multiple Orgasms Any More?

(Don't you like the "Any More" part of that question?)

Yes, some men could have more than one orgasm in a sexual "session", but this is usually younger very healthy men. There are even websites (not pornographic but informational) set up to address this designed with forums to help men achieve this phenomenon[64].

Requirements (from what I've read – no references for this):

1. You have to be very fit.

2. No pot belly – this causes all kinds of problems *plus* you don't feel very sexy when you have a belly, right?

3. Very trim and muscular (be a moderate weight lifter).

4. Perfect vitamins levels – no deficiencies.

5. Optimal (and probably natural) testosterone production and levels.

6. Great diet with optimal protein intake.

7. Preferably (but not mandatory) age less than 35 years of age.

Chapter 12

How to Really Have a Blast in Bed!

Sorry, but that's a little bit of a play on words – what I should have said was you can probably (no guarantees here) have a large semen amount if you optimize everything (see Chapter 10).

There are other supplements you can take that will help increase your semen or spermatic fluid production which leads to better and more fun orgasms for men (plus increasing the risk of getting your significant other pregnant).

Here's a current list[65]:

1. Almonds have ghrelin that helps stimulate the pituitary and essential fatty acids that assist you in making testosterone and sperm.

2. CoQ10 can increase viable sperm production[66].

3. Oysters contain zinc (important for sperm production) and dopamine (a libido enhancer).

4. Celery contains androsterone, a male perspiration hormone, which tends to turn women on.

5. Bananas contain bromelain enzyme which reverses impotence in men and riboflavin which gives men energy.

6. Avocados are from a tree the ancient Aztecs called the "testicle tree" and they contain folic acid, vitamin B6, and potassium -- all which help with sperm formation and libido.

7. Fenugreek is an herb that researchers have found can boost libido by 25% or more[67].

8. Mangoes are full of anti-oxidants -- plus they're juicy and succulent and sexy (great for foreplay).

9. Strawberries are full of anti-oxidants -- plus they're juicy and succulent and sexy (also great for foreplay).

10. Peaches are full of anti-oxidants -- plus they're juicy and succulent and sexy (also REALLY great for foreplay).

11. Figs contain lots of amino acids, which are critical for sperm production.

12. Eggs are high in protein (for sperm and tes formation) and B5 and B6 – great for libido.

13. Garlic contains allicin, which increases blood flow[68], especially beneficial for the sexual organs.

14. Liver contains cholesterol (you make testosterone from this basic building block of life) and lots of glutamine (helps with cellular energy).

No promises but these are all supposed to help.

Chapter 13

I Still Want to Father Babies, What Should I Use For Therapy?

Azoospermia is the absence of viable sperm from the spermatic fluid. Not a good thing when you want to father children.

If you're lucky you *might* have a couple of options here (I say "might" because I haven't had the chance to examine or evaluate you so I can't know for sure):

1. Is a vitamin/mineral/amino acid deficiency the root cause of your hypogonadism? Hopefully, because with Spectracell™ technology this is now a treatable cause of azoospermia or hypogonadism.

2. Is your testosterone low but your LH and FSH *not* high? Then it's Central Hypogonadism – meaning (as we've learned) your pituitary is damaged so you can't produce enough LH or FSH to stimulate your testicles to produce enough testosterone or sperm that can swim. (Of course, in my medical opinion, you have a lot more serious problems than just a low sperm count.) This is also a treatable cause of azoospermia/hypogonadism that would still allow you to father children (plus you will feel a LOT better, too).

3. Is your tes low but your LH or FSH are high? You're probably out of luck. This is Primary Hypogonadism and chances are you may have a decrease in viable sperm that prevents you from fathering children naturally.

Pretty much your only treatment option is tes cream or shots.

Vitamin/Mineral/Amino Acid Deficiency Caused-Hypogonadism

Zinc and other mineral deficiencies, or key amino acid deficiencies, I believe are the most common cause of non-traumatic hypogonadism or azoospermia. These issues have to be addressed no matter what when you're delving into the therapies for azoospermia. I always laugh when I see doctors ("fertility experts") place some young man on Clomid™ (or some other medication) to increase sperm count! I know that 1) that Clomid™ has not, nor any other oral medication (besides injectable βHCG), been shown to increase sperm count or testosterone levels, and 2) that they have not endeavored to even check testosterone levels or LH or FSH levels (the basics in my book) and certainly not a Spectracell™ (nor do they even know about it – see the section on SpectraCell™). Yet they prescribe Clomid™ or some other off the wall female fertility medication regardless of side effects or costs. Then sadly, this young man, will have his mind closed (for a while usually) to any other options as the "fertility expert" *has spoken!*

At this point I usually just keep my mouth shut. Life has a way of balancing out in the end.

Central or Pituitary Hypogonadism (remember, your doctor may call this Hypogonadotrophic Hypgonadism)

This is where your pituitary is so damaged that you cannot produce enough LH or FSH to cause your testicles to make viable sperm or testosterone. This is usually from head trauma (it can be mild trauma, or many other causes –- see Chapter 4 for more details). (Of course this can be multifactorial in causation so look at vitamin/mineral/amino acid deficiencies too!) And usually injectable βHCG is the best option here (though I will try high quality sublingual on occasion when the hypogonadism is less *severe*).

The injectable βHCG should be given subcutaneously (with little tiny insulin needles) at least 6 days a week (does not hurt to take a day off for your receptors to "recover") at a dose varying from 300 -1,500 units a day (usually at the lower end of the scale).

Most insurance companies won't pay for this (even though it's the FDA approved therapy for Hypogonadotrophic or Central Hypogonadism – ask your doctor to look in a Physician's Desk Reference® under Novarel® if he/she doubts this)(and they will), and I am not sure why -- and they usually use incredibly bogus reasons (we think you're prescribing it for a diet – huh?) to deny payment or coverage. Sad. So it's a little pricey at the pharmacy (?$175 or less? for 10,000 units) but if you shop around you can usually find it cheaper or even "compounded" (called "pre-mixed" in our area, as the compounding pharmacist pre-mixes it and then refrigerates it). You must keep it refrigerated and handle it with care as the βHCG molecule is large and incredibly fragile and not amenable to much shaking or vibration (it will go "stale" very quickly if this occurs and decline in effectiveness).

Once you start therapy on βHCG it can take 3-6 months to finally see the big increase (in libido, testosterone levels, sperm count), according to how long the testicles have set there nascent and un-stimulated.

It's critical to be patient and to be very consistent – take your HCG injections just like you're a diabetic taking insulin.

Using Clomiphene Citrate (Clomid™) – The Newest Approach

There is a better option that has been developed the last few years – using Clomiphene Citrate (Clomid™) to stimulate your own production of LH and FSH. There have been a number of studies that have shown very good results in this area at 25 mg a day[69] or even 50 mg a day, which agrees with what we've seen in our practice. It also comes in a generic so it's inexpensive. Also, according to the Sloan Kettering Institute in NYC it has minimal side effects and is very safe and effective for long-term use[70].

Clomiphene also acts as a SERM[71] (selective estrogen receptor modulator) so it blocks estrogen from negative feedback loop receptors in your hypothalamus which prevents further suppression of your luteinizing hormone (LH), which *further* increases your LH and, in the end, testosterone. This affect also lowers your testosterone/estrogen ratio, which in itself is even more beneficial according to some studies[72].

Rebooting Your LH/FSH with Clomiphene Citrate – HUH?

There is a theory that the hypothalamus (the pituitary hangs down from it) can be "rebooted" using clomiphene (yes, a hypothalamus reboot). You would have to re-activate your testicles first using βHCG for at least a few months before you start[73]. Then taking clomiphene 25-50 mg a day for 30-45 days (usually the 25 mg works just fine), and then stopping it suddenly can "reset" production in your hypothalamus[74] (causing a surge in LHRH and GnRH) and you then have a surge in your LH and FSH. This "surge" can take a few days or even a week or so but then it occasionally (not always though) happens.

– then no more long term use of HCG or even tes – you can wing it on your own!

Keep in mind this definitely is not guaranteed and does not often work but it does work.

Chapter 14

I Still Want to Father Babies, What Should I Avoid?

So you still want to father children?

Then don't take anything that will suppress your testicular or spermatic function, especially illicit drugs such as cocaine, heroin or marijuana (sorry, I know that low testosterone causes an increase in anxiety and so some have found amelioration using pot, but this does not help your tes levels or sperm count – so STOP IT!). This would include prescription steroids, testosterone (cream, gel, or shots of cypionate) and radiation therapy and certain stimulants and anti-depressants.

Also, avoid motorcycle riding, tight jeans, and trauma (bull riding?) to your testicles.

Come on! Give those "boys" a chance to produce swimmers!!! Okay?

Some Bad Things That May Kill Your Sperm

Things to avoid:

Testicular trauma (such as from playing football or being hit in the head with a baseball).

Bicycle riding – seat trauma, right?

Too tight of pants – NO SKINNY JEANS! (Okay, no one wears these anyway, right? Not now, right?)

Injection of testosterone cypionate (certainly NEVER in your testicles – but anywhere in your body).

Testosterone cream or gel will kill sperm production or at least tamp it down.

We've talked about low tes, and low vitamins, and amino acid deficiencies, but there are other things (bad things) that can cause problems with your sperm production:

Laptops on your lap (not on your desk) increases scrotal temperature – bad for sperm production.

Cell Phones -- questionable but you may not want to keep it near your groin in a pocket – studies vary but be careful.

Radiation
Duh!

But it is amazing to me that I see dentists and surgeons and radiologists and others who have some pituitary damage (so low tes and low sperm counts) from radiation exposure to their heads (or even sometimes their groins).

When you put a lead apron you should now automatically put a little lead hat on too!

Don't Let the "Boys" Get Too Hot

Just like in the laptop comment above you should know that human testes cannot function properly unless they are able to stay cooler than the rest of the body. Optimally, the male

70

anatomy is designed to create distance between the testes and the core body temperature.

If the temperature of the testicles is raised to 98° or above, sperm production ceases[75] and when production is interrupted, sperm can be negatively impacted for months afterwards.

Fevers

If you've had a virus or some kind of infectious illness that caused you to have a fever that can affect your production of viable sperm, often for months.

Briefs or Bicycle Shorts

Too tight clothing down there might cause testicles to get too close to the body raising their temperatures too high (to 98° or above again). So wear boxers if you want to conceive – leave the little boy shorts home.

Hot Tubs

Wet heat has been known for hundreds of years in India[76] as being bad for a man's testicles and causing male impotence.

"The wet heat method has been known since the 4th century B.C. It involves placing the testes in hot water (116 degrees Fahrenheit) for 45 minutes every night for 3 weeks. This provides protection for 6 months."

Varicose Veins of the Testes (Varicoceles)

Approximately 15 percent of men have varicoceles, or enlarged varicose veins in the scrotum, usually in the left testicle. When a man is experiencing a low sperm count, doctors may recommend varicocele repair, a procedure that repairs enlarged varicose veins in the scrotum surgically or via percutaneous embolization, a nonsurgical procedure using a catheter.

This causes an unobstructive azoospermia.

"Although there is no conclusive evidence that a varicocele repair improves spontaneous pregnancy rates, varicocelectomy improves sperm parameters (count and total and progressive motility), reduces sperm DNA damage and seminal oxidative stress, and improves sperm ultramorphology. The various methods of repair are all viable options, but microsurgical repair seems to be associated with better outcomes[77]."

Obesity

Compared to normal and overweight men, obese fertile men have reduced testicular function and significantly lower sperm counts. Although obesity reduces sperm count, only extreme levels of obesity may negatively influence male reproductive potential[78].

A Party Lifestyle

Tobacco, alcohol, and marijuana can impair sexual function and sperm quality.

Alcohol abuse negatively affects semen quality and production, while cigarette smoking impairs sperm's motility, accord.

"Heavy smoking was associated with decreased sperm counts and alcohol consumption was associated with increased numbers of morphologically abnormal sperm[79]."

Marijuana isn't safe either. Smoking pot has been shown to reduce sperm count, sperm function, and overall male fertility[80].

More Trouble for Sperm

Blockages of the testes can negatively affect sperm production (whether by a birth defect, infection, trauma, or vasectomy, a blockage might prevent the sperm from entering the semen).

Genetic disorders also can be a problem – such as Klinefelter's Syndrome or cystic fibrosis are the most common.

"Klinefelter's syndrome (KS) is one the most common sex chromosomal abnormalities and is characterized by hypergonadotropic hypogonadism and infertility. Some men with non-mosaic syndrome have azoospermia and only few have oligospermia[81]."

"Most men with CF[82] have significant anatomical abnormalities of the reproductive tract causing infertility..."

Other detrimental factors such as anti-sperm antibodies, testicular cancer, undescended testicles, and many other things can affect sperm. So make sure a knowledgeable physician takes the time to examine you down there if needed.

Chapter 15

Why Is βHCG (Beta Human Chorionic Gonadotropin) 3D for Male Infertility Issues?

Unlike topical or injectable testosterone (which *only* increase your testosterone level), βHCG will increase your:

1. Testosterone production from your Leydig cells (via the 80% LH portion of the βHCG molecule).

2. Spermatozoa production from your Sertoli cells (via the 20% FSH portion of the βHCG molecule).

3. Libido via all the functions of the βHCG molecule.

This is why daily injectable **βHCG is the most natural therapy** out there for central (pituitary, also called *hypogonadotrophic*) hypogonadism and is FDA approved for this purpose. (Remember, it will not work for primary or testicular hypgonadism.)

But you have to be consistent and get the dose right (everyone's a "snowflake" and seems to require different therapies and doses – so you have to be patient). And give it time – you were not broken yesterday so I cannot get you better tomorrow.

So is βHCG perfect and wonderful?

No.

Clearly none of these can make you perform exactly like you were originally designed to work – medicine and our therapies are just not that good yet. I have to explain this all the time to people. Clearly, as a profession we are *very* limited. We are not super doctors like you see on television, and we can never make you perfect again, so at best I can get you a ways beyond just functional.

But for a lot that's a miracle and pretty awesome.

But not perfect for most.

Can't do it.

Maybe I can get some to 98% on a really good day.

So for now, it is the best we have. And that's a long way from the alternatives

Chapter 16

Compounded Testosterone Creams vs Testosterone Gels

Sorry to the manufacturer of the prescription (as seen on TV) big pharma gels, but I've never seen them work. I believe this is actually more through selection by the patient (meaning *if* it's working for them, and their doctor prescribed it, why would they quit it, and bother finding me as I am pretty much invisible? And if it's not working then they get disgusted and find me or some other alternative) than actually a bad design of product, but it's still my perception.

I have had very good results with a well compounded lipodermal cream (MedQuest® in Utah is one of the biggest compounding pharmacies in the world and make a really good quality cream) or lipodermal gel (Central Drug® in La Habra, California is run by a smart group of pharmacology doctorates who teach at USC medical school and their compounded gel is awesome), plus many others. Though some compounded cream/gels are pretty awful so be smart and try another pharmacy if the cream/gel you have does not work – your doctor will have to approve this new script, of course.

Problems With The Topical Testosterone?

Yes. After "poor absorption" issues, the biggest problem is "transference." (This can occur with both the gels and the creams.)

Transference is where you have a tes cream or gel on and hug your wife or daughter, or go to bed with it on, and it gets all over your sheets, then all over your wife or daughter or son, who then end up with *really* high testosterone levels. That's a problem (not if it occurs short term but certainly if it goes on for months and months or years). Okay?

For example: I saw a very successful business woman in a consult a few years ago where she was suffering from abnormally high levels of testosterone. She'd been to numerous physicians, including the Mayo Clinic in Arizona, with no luck. No one could figure it out. They had MRI'd her and CAT scanned her and ultra sounded her ovaries, drawn gallons of blood, all to no avail. They were all scratching their heads and her last big expert had suggested a hysterectomy (?!?!?!?!) because he could think of nothing else (I guess even PCOS had not crossed his mind, but that's for another day). After, I heard all of this I just asked her if her husband used a topical testosterone, and she said yes. To her dumbfounded look I just said have him wipe it off with a baby wipe before he gets in bed or hugs you or the kids, and make sure when you get home you wash all your beddings.

It worked.

This was just a simple and obvious case of topical tes transference. To this day she thanks me whenever she sees me or if I'm in her area speaking.

Chapter 17

Plan D: Injectable Testosterone

There are several forms of legally available injectable testosterone – cypionate (cheapest and most readily available), enanthate, and even propionate (must be compounded).

And to be clear, I am slowly becoming a big fan of injectable testosterone cypionate.

It's cheap.

It's once a week of a few seconds of pain to take (it's a shot given intramuscularly with an inch long needle – not as bad as it sounds).

And it ALWAYS works (at least as far as optimizing your testosterone levels -- often it's too good and we have to back it off somewhat).

Every doctor can prescribe according to how they see things but for me to help the average patient keep a stable, optimal, happy level of testosterone (I can only affect the TOTAL testosterone level not the more important FREE level which is really more determined on the ever mysterious SHBG or Sex Hormone Binding Globulin) I need to have them take (on average) approximately 1 cc (or ml or milliliter) intramuscularly every week on the same day. This works fairly well for most guys.

I do see a lot of physicians who give the shot once a month or at best every two weeks. Let me tell you what this feels like –

you feel great for about 5-6 days then you slowly enter depressive, fatigued HELL until you get your next shot (be it 8-9 or 22-26 days later). I would not do this to my dog.

I've already shown where the literature, and the preventive medicine community, says a normal level of TOTAL testosterone is 800-1200 ng/dl – so why not keep them there?

I know of no reason not to, as we keep diabetic patients receiving insulin at an optimal blood sugar and HbA1C when we're able. This makes for healthier and happier patients (and a LOT of my patients are physicians and you want them happy, right?) plus they live a lot longer, our real goal.

Are There Other Injectable Testosterone Options?

Sure -- testosterone enanthate and testosterone deaconate, or propionate – a rare few of my patients ask for these hoping to get better results but I just haven't seen it.

Others are harder to find or require a special DEA capability I do not have nor do I wish to request.

And I don't care what you read on the internet – it does not make it legal. Or beneficial for you to take.

(Have I scared you off yet? For you that will ask, I have a very full and tiny practice, with many of my patients being physicians. I did not and am not writing this book to attract new patients, instead I am writing to help doctors and patients deal with their doctors [or themselves] to give and get good therapy supported by the literature. I only see 4-8 patients a day at most, and have a busy life and like to take care of myself and my family in a healthy way. Thanks for understanding.)

Chapter 18

Natural Therapies That May Help Elevate Testosterone Levels?

We talked about a lot of natural vitamins and amino acids and why they work. Let me review a few.

L-Arginine

L-Arginine at approximately 3,000 mg a day has been shown to increase testosterone levels and reduce vascular inflammation (or is that a cause of the increased testosterone) and help with viable sperm production. And I especially like the Pro-Argi-9™ that's out there (again I am not paid, nor am I distributor, nor am I a consultant for the company that makes this supplement – I just think it's really good).

Complete Amino Acid Supplements

Another amino acid supplement that I have been suggesting and that's fairly new on the market is Laminine™, another MLM product that's really excellent (again, I am not paid, nor am I distributor, nor am I a consultant for the company that makes this supplement – it's just really good). It is a COMPLETE amino acid supplement (meaning it has all 43 amino acids in one capsule) so when I get someone with an amino acid deficiency or two upon Spectracell™ testing I have to assume they might have others (the Spectracell™ Comprehensive test, as good as it is, is only able to look at only seven amino acids currently) beyond the scope or ability of *anyone* to test. So I often now suggest adding Laminine™ to their supplement list and I've seen some pretty amazing things happen which makes me believe that there are amino acid deficiencies causing disease states out there that are just not diagnosed.

(If you're interested in this product, and can't find anyone in your area that distributes this, call my office in Lindon, Utah and talk to Mindi, my front desk manager. Because of my consulting business I am not signed up for any products so I ask Mindi to.)

Fish Oil

When I mention fish oil here I am really talking about the DHA portion (which is the most beneficial for testosterone and sperm production AND cardiovascular and joint health).

We know from several studies that there is a minimum of the DHA (docosahexanoic acid) and EPA (eicosapentanoic acid) you must intake each day for optimum cardiovascular and sexual health.

This amount is 2,500 milligrams (mg) per day.

If you read the *back* of the bottle (not the front) of fish oil you will see (it's a recent FDA requirement) the amount of EPA and DHA per dose or per capsule (make sure you differentiate this) and so do the math so this number equals 2,500 milligrams and that's how many capsules you should take. (You may have to work up to this number slowly if you tend to burp up fish oil -- start low, go slow, and give it a few weeks or months for your body to get there.) Note that if you have had cardiovascular disease (a stroke, or angina, an MI, or heart disease) you should be on 5,000 mg a day of the DHA and EPA.

Currently I am taking two different fish oils every day, and here they are and why I take them:

1. Source Naturals™ Omega-3 High Potency Formula® Fish Oil from www.vitacost.com. This very high quality yet inexpensive fish oil is both **pharmaceutical grade** (one of my requirements) and **molecularly distilled** (another requirement) and at 850 mg of DHA+EPA per capsule, you only need to take 3 a day to reach your minimum 2,500 mg/day of the EPA and the DHA. This is almost as good as the very expensive prescription fish oil that's out there. (I take 3 a day of these.)

2. There's also a new product made by Young Living Essential Oils™ whose design I had some input in (though we do not make it for nor do I profit from the sales of it in any way) the design. It contains both DHA at (the best part of the fish oil component), Vitamin D3 (the cholecalciferol version – the best), and CoQ10 (in the form of ubiquinol, the most easily absorbed and most potent Co-Enzyme Q10 – by 8X *[hat tip to Dr Scott Johnson, Educational Director at Young Living Essential Oils, LLC]*). It also contains clove and German chamomile and spearmint. It's an excellent cardiovascular and adult health capsule, and Gary Young and Marc Schreuder at Young Living did a great job in pulling it off. (I take 2 a day of these.)

What else is in this recently new product?

"Clove has antiseptic qualities, contains high amounts of eugenol for the body's natural defenses and regulates the body's natural response to stress.

82

German chamomile- this oil contains chamazulene, a compound that helps our body's natural inflammatory response.

Spearmint- spearmint aids digestion and supports respiratory health.

In addition, CoQ10 is also added to [*this product*]. Young Living uses bioidentical Kaneka Q10 that is the highest quality CoQ10 in the world. CoQ10 is also known as ubiquinone. It is a natural oil-soluble substance essential for health. CoQ10 helps normal function of the body's cells.

D3 is also found in [*this product*]. D3 helps with normal circulation, mood and the body's ability to absorb calcium.

A bottle of [*this product*] contains DHA-rich fish oils, clove oil, German chamomile oil, spearmint oil, CoQ10 and D3. These ingredients were added to give the overall benefits of general wellness including brain, heart, eye and joint health[83]."

"[*This product*] provides more than 300mg of beneficial DHA and 135 mg of EPA per serving per 4 liquid capsules[84]."

SOMETHING REALLY REALLY NEW

Something else that's all natural that might be able to help men have uhhh more "energy" at those key moments in their lives has now been found. As you know I am involved as a consultant with Young Living™ Essential Oils in their Research and Discovery department and in the last year, Gary Young suggested I test a specific oil (obtained from a tree grown in the far north mountains) and was really shocked by what I saw. This had a dramatic effect on male "energy" across the board with everyone (small number at the time admittedly but the jump was significant) that I had apply it topically. It was a real natural booster. It was like Gary (and I – but this is clearly his company and I was just lucky enough to help him confirm his great intuition about this) had found the Holy Grail for these kind of nutraceuticals and it looks to be really cool (maybe 'hot" would be a better adjective). The current FDA and DEA rules and environment constrain me from saying anything more about this but looks to be a superior natural men's energy booster. Working with the R&D team at YLEO (Cole Woolley, PhD, Rich Carlson, PhD, and Rex Kidman) of course led by Gary Young, we're trying to make it into a men's cologne that smells really sexy (our plan is to come out with a woman's *eau de toilette* version later this year). This one should be really fun and huge product for all men to try. I love it. This product will be ready to go to market in July or August of 2013 (and I think YLEO distributors are about to be very happy with this one) so look for a Young Living distributor near you and get that fish oil/D3 product and this new men's "cologne" product – you won't be sorry. (And Full AMA Disclosure rules says you should know that I will probably be helping with and profiting from the manufacturing of this product – so please try it, see how your energy does, and then buy twelve more bottles – I have 4 kids in college.)

Chapter 19

What Other Therapies Should I Consider Besides Testosterone?

I think we've covered a huge plethora of other supplements which you could take that might help with your sexuality (instead of guessing just remember to get a SpectraCell™ Comprehensive Panel before you start). So let's review some other options:

Exercise

Weight Lifting – helps with fitness and also causes release of all kinds of cool hormones that help your libido.

Yoga – stretching and relaxing never hurts, and looking at hot girls around you doing the same can't either.

Lots of **practice** (in the bedroom)

Eating a **proper diet**

Eating "good" fats (such as in avocados)

Chapter 20

Will Taking Testosterone Increase My PSA or Risk of Prostate Cancer?

Taking testosterone used to be thought of as something that would increase your risk of developing prostate cancer or that it would elevate your PSA – but now we know that this is definitely not the case. There have been numerous studies, which have shown that higher testosterone levels (high normal or optimal) can dramatically reduce your risk of developing prostate cancer or prostate cancer recurrence.

"When the patients were divided into normal- and low- sTT (serum Total Testosterone) level groups according to testosterone value (300 ng/dl), the probability of detecting prostate cancer was 3.3-fold higher in hypogonadal men as compared with eugonadal men[85]."

Wow! **330% increase in prostate cancer rates in men with historically low testosterone.**

Men, GET YOUR TESTOSTERONE LEVELS UP TO NORMAL!

Chapter 21

Are There Other Health Reasons to Do All of This?

The short answer is of course YES.

Optimized testosterone levels cause so many good things to occur that it's AMAZING! Most of these things I've already covered but here they are with the research referenced on each:

[From my Program120 textbook]

What optimized testosterone levels can give your male patients:

1. Decreases endothelial resistance acting as a potent vasodilator[86].

2. Higher total testosterone and SHBG (sex hormone binding globulin) levels are inversely related to carotid atherosclerosis, suggesting their potential importance in reducing atherosclerotic risk in postmenopausal women not using HRT[87].

3. Higher free testosterone levels in men are associated with higher ejection fractions (higher cardiac output)[88].

4. Age, HDL, and **free testosterone** may be stronger predictors of degree of coronary artery disease than are blood pressure, cholesterol, diabetes, smoking, and body mass index (BMI)[89].

5. Despite the literature replete with supporting studies[90] [91], cardiologists continue to ignore the favorable benefits of natural testosterone replacement. Don't do the same.

6. There is evidence to suggest that low concentrations of testosterone are associated with an increased risk of CVD in men[92].

7. Testosterone concentration is inversely correlated with procoagulable factors, plasminogen activator inhibitor, and fibrinogen[93]. Give enough testosterone to obtain a good physiologic level and these coagulation factors decline.

8. Testosterone, at physiologic concentrations, induces coronary artery dilation and increases coronary blood flow in men with established coronary artery disease[94].

9. Normal physiological levels improve insulin resistance by bolstering the functionality of insulin receptors[95]. (Also, see Chapter 6 Diabetes and see Chapter 8 Alzheimer's Disease). There is an association in men between low concentrations of free and total testosterone and hyperinsulinemia[96].

10. Normal physiological levels increases muscle mass[97].

11. Lower levels predispose to increased BMI and diabetes[98].

12. Normal physiological levels prevents Alzheimer's disease. Low levels of testosterone are an independent risk factor[99]! (See Chapter 8 Alzheimer's Disease)

13. Normal physiological levels prevents osteoporosis in men and women by increasing bone mineral density (BMD)[100].

14. Normal physiological levels improves erectile dysfunction in men[101].

15. Normal physiological levels improves libido and well-being in men and women (in women who have undergone oophorectomy and hysterectomy, transdermal testosterone improves sexual function and psychological well-being[102] *[Author-- as reported in the New England Journal of Medicine using optimized levels from younger women who were menstruating, confirming once again our repeated observation that the peer reviewed studies use the optimized levels and so should the practitioners]*).

16. In adult males, testosterone maintains muscle mass and strength, fat distribution, bone mass, erythropoiesis, male hair pattern, libido and potency, and spermatogenesis[103].

17. Testosterone increases HGH production in the elderly -- it is critical to create that rich hormonal milieu or stew that allows all eight cylinders of your patient's hormone engines to fire properly. In light of a Mayo Clinic study having shown that giving hypogonadal men, especially elderly men, testosterone causes them to also increase production of endogenous HGH[104]. This is awesome and a heck of a lot cheaper then giving rHGH!

18. 35% of heart patients treated with testosterone *improved* by at least one NYHA (New York Heart Association) class[105].

19. Testosterone replacement therapy improves functional capacity and symptoms in men with moderately severe heart failure[106]. *[Why don't cardiologists put all of their patients on this? – Program 120® Editor]*

20. Testosterone can dramatically improve endurance especially in the frail elderly[107] (but really since it will build muscle and bone mass this can occur at almost any level from age 40 years on[108]).

21. Sex hormones play a key role in numerous physiologic processes and functions and clearly impact wound healing in the all ages of patients[109] but especially the elderly[110].

22. Maintaining appropriate levels until death allows improved cognition, better affect, more rapid thinking/processing skills[111] and decision making and better muscle mass[112].

23. With your erectile dysfunction patients don't ever give Viagra® until you have worked them up for hypogonadism or testosterone deficiency[113]. Experience shows you will often need to give both testosterone[114] and sildenafil (or your favorite phosphodiesterase inhibitor) to more adequately treat some ED cases.

24. Testosterone in patients can not only improve insulin resistance but increase the number and health of insulin receptors[115]. First, the lack of testosterone in men has been strongly associated with metabolic syndrome[116]. Second, giving testosterone to these men can help clear up the insulin resistance and absolve the pre-diabetic stage[117].

25. Testosterone improves vascular resistance, reduces systolic blood pressure[118], improves dyslipidemias[119] (lowers triglycerides, raises HDL), and improves cardiac output.

26. Normal physiological levels causes improvement in osteoporosis[120] as is clear in a number of studies[121].

27. Testosterone in hypogonadal men improves Alzheimer's disease (see Alzheimer's Chapter), Multiple Sclerosis (MS)[122], Huntington's disease[123], Parkinson's disease, and others. As a matter of fact, testosterone loss may be a risk factor for cognitive decline and possibly for dementia[124] and is clearly neuroprotective[125] and exogenous supplementation proved beneficial for cognitive and brain function in elderly men.

28. Testosterone supplementation can increase red blood cells, an extremely beneficial factor for most older men *and women*, causing a relative erythrocytosis. Do not be mistaken – this is not a polycythemia or a polycythemia vera (see below) – this is just a beneficial eyrthrocytosis that deserves no treatment, and even minimal observation[126]. Most men *and women* who are hypogonadal are also anemic[127] and supplementing them with testosterone can often resolve this.

29. Testosterone replacement therapy (TRT) improves lower urinary tract symptoms in men (LUTS – urinary frequency, urgency, halting or residual urine in the bladder, etc) and shrinks BPH. Erectile dysfunction (ED), which is absolutely associated with hypogonadisim or low levels of testosterone, has now been associated with LUTS[128] and BPH[129].

30. In women, testosterone is the main hormone that prevents urogenital and vaginal atrophy – save your female patients from decades of dry vaginas, poor sex lives and embarrassing stress

incontinence by giving them a little testosterone just like their ovaries did!

31. Testosterone decline with aging in men is associated with osteoarthritis development[130] and worsening rheumatoid arthritis[131].

32. Testosterone Replacement Therapy (TRT), unlike what is commonly believed, is NOT associated with causing frank PIN (prostate intraepithelial neoplasia) to become full prostate cancer. After 1 year of TRT men with PIN treated at Beth Israel Deaconess Medical Center at the Harvard Medical School do NOT have a greater increase in PSA or a significantly increased risk of cancer than men without PIN. These results indicate that TRT is not contraindicated in men with a history of PIN[132].

33. Contrary to what your local cardiologist says (and some papers erroneously claim as a side effect) physiological testosterone replacement did not adversely affect blood coagulation status (plasminogen activator inhibitor-1 (PAI-1), fibrinogen, tissue plasminogen activator (tPA) and full blood count)[133].

34. Low levels of testosterone in elderly men increase fall risk by 40%[134] (probably secondary to weaker antigravity and balance muscles). Fall risk was higher in men with lower bioavailable testosterone levels. The effect of testosterone level was independent of poorer physical performance, suggesting that the effect of testosterone on fall risk may be mediated by other androgen actions.

Chapter 22

I've Had Prostate Cancer, am I Doomed?

Prostate cancer is very common and for your years it was thought that years of high testosterone caused it.

Nothing could be further from the truth.

We now know from years of really well done studies that it's actually years of low testosterone that causes the increased risk of prostate cancer[135].

But after you've been surgerized and had your prostate removed, received your chemo, and are cleared by your doctors, the current research shows that *within a month* you should be receiving testosterone replacement therapy.

This aggressive therapy helps prevent depression, cardiovascular disease and other hypogonadism related diseases.

"Thus, testosterone therapy is effective and, while followed by a rise in prostate specific antigen, does not appear to increase cancer recurrence rates, even in men with high-risk prostate cancer. However, given the retrospective nature of this and prior studies, testosterone therapy in men with history of prostate cancer should be undertaken with a vigorous surveillance protocol[136]."

From my favorite urologist at Harvard: "Although no controlled studies have been performed to date to document the safety of testosterone therapy in men with prostate cancer, the limited available evidence suggests that such treatment may not pose an undue risk of prostate cancer recurrence or progression[137]."

Chapter 23

I've Had Testicular Cancer, am I Doomed?

Testicular cancer occurs after cells in your testicle become malignant and start going crazy, multiplying like mad. They usually do not produce testosterone.

Are there different types of testicular cancer?

Yes.

"Most (95%) testicular cancer originates in undeveloped cells (germ cells) that produce sperm. These tumors, called germ cell tumors (GCTs), are most common in men between the ages of 20 and 40 and are **curable in more than 95% of cases**. There are two main types: seminomas and nonseminomas. A third type, called stromal tumors, develops in the supporting tissues of the testicle.

Approximately 40% of GCTs are seminomas, which are classified as either typical or spermatocytic. Typical seminomas account for 90% of this type. They **often cause unilateral (i.e., on one side) testicle enlargement or more often a painless lump in the testicle**. Spermatocytic seminomas grow slowly, usually do not spread to other parts of the body (metastasize), and are most common around age 65.

Nonseminomas account for 60% of GCTs and develop in younger men (usually between 15 and 35). Most nonseminomas contain cells from at least two subtypes, including the following:

- Choriocarcinoma (rare; aggressive; likely to metastasize)

- Embryonal carcinoma (accounts for 20% of cases; likely to metastasize)
- Teratoma (usually benign in children; rarely metastasize)
- Yolk sac carcinoma (most common in young boys; rare in men)

Testicular cancer may also develop in the supportive, hormone-producing tissue of the testicles (stroma). This type accounts for 4% of testicular cancer in men and 20% in boys. Types of stromal tumors include Leydig cell tumors and Sertoli cell tumors[138]." [Thank you University of Miami]

Read that last paragraph again – only 4% of testicular cancers in men (20% in boys) produce an overabundance of testosterone.

For some reasons many physicians mistakenly confuse high normal levels of exogenous testosterone with causation of testicular cancer -- *these physicians think that testosterone is a cause of, and not an effect of, testosterone.*

It is not.

High normal testosterone taken exogenously suppresses your testicular cells, and does not stimulate them. It does not cause cancer and if anything, this prevents testicular cancer.

So no, you are not doomed.

And if you've had and survived (most likely) and testicular cancer, receiving testosterone from exogenous sources (say -- your doctor) will not increase your risk of occurrence, but actually decrease your risk.

Plus normalizing and optimizing your testosterone levels will also decrease your risk of depression, heart attack, stroke and other cancers (see the next few chapters).

Chapter 24

I've had a Heart Attack, am I Doomed?

It's bad; no doubt about it IF you've had an MI, so you have to do everything that you can to prevent it from ever reoccurring. That said, anything, and I mean *anything*, you do to improve your vascular status and reduce your risks of a heart recurrence will almost always help your love life and your libido.

If it were my body or you were my brother (or patient) here's what I'd tell you (and then we'll go to what I would do to help):

Optimize your serum testosterone levels, and do it as naturally as possible. Why? Normal or optimized testosterone levels will reduce vascular inflammation[139]. Optimizing testosterone levels will also lower your blood pressure[140], normalize your weight[141], and usually reduce your cholesterol levels[142].

Plus it also reduces depression[143].

If possible also start a plaque regression program.

Uhh, what?

I said a plaque regression program – that's where you make plaque go away or melt away out of your arteries. The theory being (not much of a theory since it's undoubtedly true in 99.8% of cases of myocardial infarction) that if you have plaque in your coronary arteries you'll have plaque in your penile arteries making erections more difficult (or as some call it – ED or erectile dysfunction).

There are six known things that cause plaque regression (these are known from really well done and now confirmed studies – I know this because I lecture on this cool little subject all over the world):

A. Niacin 2000 mg a day can cause regression[144]. Wow, watch out for the hideous flushing you will have at this dose and you really have to work up to this amount.
B. Simvastatin 80 mg/day[145] or rosuvastatin 80 mg/day[146] – these are the only two statins that will do this but they will melt the plaque away but only at this dose. You also must make darn sure you take high doses of CoQ10 at these doses and that you get your LFTs (liver function tests checked regularly like every 3 months).
C. Keeping or getting your Free T3 (thyroid measurement for those of you with low thyroid functionality) around 4.0 ng/dl can lead to plaque regression[147]. This can be touchy because too high a T3 level or T4 level and your heart will beat too hard and then you will possibly get another heart attack and die – so be *careful* with this one.
D. Actos™ (pioglitazone) is amazing at causing plaque regression[148] but are the potential side effects worth it (i.e. bladder cancer[149])? You'll have to decide (I've taken myself for a total of 6 months – minimal if any risk).
E. Optimizing your IGF-1 levels will also cause plaque regression[150]. So go see a good anti-aging physician or a good pituitary endocrinologist (really hard to find).
F. A blood pressure maintained below 120/70 will prevent or cause plaque regression[151]. It must be done properly using a stepwise approach involving centrally acting blood pressure meds (such as lisinopril, hydrochlorothiazide, Micardis™ or amlodipine).

Enroll In a Cardiac Rehab Program and Stick To It! (Get in shape! But do it RIGHT!)

A good Cardiac Rehab program will have you exercise usually in your local hospital in a stepwise approach, while they have physical therapists and technicians there to monitor you closely. This is critical so you don't have a recurrence of the MI and you can take things nice and gradually.

Chapter 25

I've Got Migraines, Should I Take Testosterone?

Yes, you should definitely take testosterone for chronic male migraine-type or severe headaches.

Why?

Migraine headaches in men (but not women) are almost all caused by low testosterone, especially the cluster type[152] – this lack of testosterone causes a vascular inflammation which is most acutely felt in the very sensitive arteries or vessels in the head. This is why migraines are a risk factor for future strokes – the severe vascular inflammation[153] is what causes the risk.

In almost all cases normalizing testosterone makes the severity and frequency of the migraine headaches decline or even go away. This may not happen right away and might take a month or two but eventually they do – my rule is to get rid of them completely (or I feel like I'm doing something wrong). Now you can see why nearly all of my patients get off their pain meds within the first year – they don't need them.

This is a far happier option than Imetrex®[154] or narcotics.

Chapter 26

I've Had A Stroke, Am I Doomed?

No, you're not doomed.

Strokes are scary and horrible. They are almost all caused by some form of chronic vascular inflammation.

Vascular inflammation can be and is caused, as I've said numerous times throughout this book, by low testosterone levels. Think of testosterone as a lubricating oil that keeps everything smooth and slick, especially arteries.

In my mind I think regarding doctors who say no to this therapy are like doctors who would not treat a broken leg on a diabetic.

So why not?

Even if they are physically unable to have sex, optimizing testosterone not only makes the man feel better overall but also reduces his risk for stroke recurrence by reducing vascular inflammation[155].

We know now (remember, I helped author a textbook on preventive medicine) from the modern literature that once a stroke occurs EVERYTHING possible should be done to recover and prevent recurrence.

Here's some of what you can and should do to prevent recurrence (get my **Program 120 Handbook A or Program 120 textbook** for more info):

"First a Note on Previous Stroke

In a study performed in Australia of over 10 years of follow-up with patients, the risk of first recurrent stroke was found to be six times greater (43%) than the risk of first-ever stroke in the general population of the same age and sex, with almost one half of survivors remain disabled, and one seventh requiring institutional care .

The rule as a physician who cares about prevention is to treat these stroke survivors MUCH more aggressively and exactly – bring everything to bear.

1. **Hypogonadism (low testosterone levels in older males) = Increased Arterial Stiffness and Increased Stroke Risk!** Free Testosterone Index (i.e. free testosterone level blood levels) in one study in London showed a strong positive relationship with Systemic Arterial Compliance (i.e. arterial stiffness) concluding that the known association between lower androgenicity and increased cardiovascular risk in men might be explained by altered vascular stiffness[156].

2. **Lack of testosterone (hypogonadism) causes all kinds of vascular problems!** A population-based cohort study conducted in 1995 amongst 141 Swedish men born in 1944 now with an abnormal hormone secretion pattern were found to have an elevated mean arterial pressure, fasting insulin and insulin:glucose ratio (hyperinsulinemia) compared with men with a normal secretion pattern[157]. *[Ah ha, this proves hypogonadism causes metabolic syndrome too—Program 120® ed]*

3. **Consequences of the chronic hypogonadal state include** progressive insulin resistance (insulin receptor failure) which leads to a high triglyceride-low HDL pattern of dyslipidemia and increased cardiovascular risk. All of these factors eventually contribute to the **CHAOS Complex:** coronary disease, hypertension, adult-onset diabetes mellitus, obesity and/or stroke as permanent changes unfold. Other problems stemming

from hypogonadism include osteopenia, extreme fatigue, depression, insomnia, loss of aggressiveness and erectile dysfunction all of which develop over variable periods of time[158].

4. **Chronic hypothyroidism increases the risk of stroke** - it is reported to be one of the causes of hypertension or elevated cholesterol levels, the established risk factors of stroke[159].

5. **Hypothyroidism is worse than Hyperthyroidism.** Hyperthyroidism is associated with atrial fibrillation and cardioembolic stroke. Hypothyroidism is associated with a worse cardiovascular risk factor profile and leads to progression of atherosclerosis[160] (and stroke).

More Details:

Stroke Prevention

Generally, anything you can do for your patients (as detailed in the cardiovascular chapter) to lower their cardiovascular risk factors will dramatically reduce their risk of stroke. Quit smoking, lower their cholesterol, watch their diet and lose weight, lower their blood pressure to the 120/70 range, get on a statin, get on an aspirin as suggested, protect their brain from injury (studies have shown that a closed head injury can increase your risk for further head trauma by 4 fold and increase your risk of Alzheimer's disease by 75% so protect your brain and the brains of those you love) and get on fish oil.

The rule is protect their brain by protecting their heart.

1. Aspirin for Primary Stroke Prevention

Generally at risk (but they are in the low risk strata) individuals should take 325 mgm/day of aspirin. This is especially true if they are less than 65 years of age and have atrial fibrillation with no other risk factors.

If your patient does not have atrial fibrillation and no contraindications then they should take an 81 mgm enteric coated aspirin a day. Aspirin significantly reduced the risk of major cardiovascular events, ischemic stroke, and myocardial infarction among women 65 years of age or older[161].

Remember, that in Chapter 1 we advised an aspirin protocol half way between these two positions -- half an adult aspirin every day in the afternoon.

2.Exercise (Fast Walking) and Lower Stress (Remember 1-4-7 FITT®)

Exercise in the prevention of stroke is oddly debated in this field. Let's look at some studies and known benefits of exercise.

When hypertensive subjects not suffering from obesity (Body Mass Index < 30) already under pharmacological therapy were studied, the majority (168 out of 189) performed a six-week program of mobility exercise based on fast walking (defined in studies as > 4 mph), leading to a decrease in their mean 24 h systolic blood pressures from 143.1 to 135.5 mmHg and a decrease in their mean 24 h diastolic blood pressure from 91.1 to 84.8 mmHg[162], numbers that clearly dramatically reduce their relative risk for stroke.

With that said a large review study showed that recreational and occupational physical activity were both associated with some reduction in risk of stroke[163]. So tell your patients just to get off the sofa and go out and do something, even if it is fun!

In the best retrospective review and assessment done to date of exercise and stroke risk the researchers concluded that exercise causes definite beneficial modification of major stroke risk factors such as hypertension, cardiovascular disease, insulin resistance/diabetes, obesity; and asserts favorable effects on conditions that worsen stroke risk such as atherosclerosis, endothelial dysfunction, hypercoagulability; and exercise reduces harmful biomarkers/risk factors such as platelet activity/aggregation, fibrinogen Triglycerides Inflammatory markers (WBC count, CRP) Plasma viscosity Coagulation factors (VIII, IX, vWF); and leads to an increase of beneficial factors such as t-PA activity, HDL, insulin sensitivity' and lipoprotein lipase (decreases lipoprotein(a)). The majority of the studies they reviewed also showed decided benefits to physical activity and stroke risk reduction[164].

Remember 1-4-7 FITT® from Chapter 13 – that's 1 hour a day, 4 mph, 7 days a week to get these results.

The Program 120® team believes that exercise inarguably decreases the risk of stroke as it does all cardiovascular disease and to think otherwise is nonsense. We also believe that daily consistent healthy exercise will reduce your stress and hypercoagulability.

3. Reduce Hypertension (Especially Early Morning)

Early treatment with lifestyle modification

For early treatment, the studies such as JNC-7 are supportive[165], so start now and treat your patients at the prehypertensive stage (120-139/80-89) with aggressive lifestyle modification which includes minimizing dietary sodium to less than 2.4 g per day; increasing exercise to at least 30 minutes per day, four days per week (at a minimum); limiting alcohol consumption to two drinks or less per day for men and one drink or less per day for women; following the Dietary Approaches to Stop Hypertension (DASH) eating plan (high in fruits, vegetables, potassium, calcium, and magnesium; low in fat and salt); and achieving a weight loss goal of 10 lb. (4.5 kg) or more[166]. The Program 120® team advises a more aggressive approach such as exercising one hour per day at 4 mph for seven days a week (1-4-7), living as salt free as possible (except for as needed by exercise demands), and following a lifestyle such as the Zone® or a combined DASH/low sodium lifestyle or diet[167] which is effective in nearly 80% of patients studied who complied (and this was for patients not with just prehypertension but with full Stage I hypertension).

Bring both systolic and diastolic blood pressure levels in your patients under complete control – clearly the studies show this will reduce their mortality, especially later in life.

We're going to leap over the current recommendations from JNC-7 [168]for Type I and Type II Hypertension and advise that, whether your patient has compelling reasons (diabetes, CAD, CKD, etc) or not, you should carefully bring their blood pressure down to below 120/70 or thereabouts.

Let's put that BP goal in big numbers so you never ever forget it:

******BP GOAL → 120/70******

However, do it slowly, and make sure their blood pressure does not go too low and that they do not get light headed. To achieve this you can and should use multiple medications to make sure their blood pressure control is "perfect" though an ACE or ARB (i.e. telmisartan) as part of the mix are very much indicated.

When a medication is necessary

Many questions should now present themselves...

Will this patient require multiple medications for blood pressure control?

Will an ARB such as telmisartan (Micardis®) work alone or do we need something else?

One medication such as telmisartan would be great if it worked to control the BP properly, and if it does – fine. But we know from the ALLHAT study that multiple medications are necessary for the majority (60%) of patients with hypertension[169]. We advise that you pull the landmark ALLHAT study and article as footnoted and review it thoroughly.

But if you treat your patients more aggressively at earlier stages in their lives maybe they will never get to the point that they need two or more BP meds to control their hypertension?

Why Telmisartan?

The ARB, telmisartan (Micardis®, Priotor®) not only reduces blood pressure more than adequately for the majority of younger patients but it does a number of other critical things such as reducing or ending microproteinuria (renal protection), reduces endothelial inflammation (vascular protection), plus potent 24 hour protection, and weight loss (shrinks adipose cells) while not causing ED or impotence (actually improves ED),and reducing proteinuria.

106

Telmisartan has a particularly interesting profile for stroke; given the 24-hour efficacy with more pronounced protection against the morning blood pressure surge and peroxisome proliferator-activated receptor-gamma activity at clinical doses. (Micardis®/Priotor®)

4. Lose Weight

Weight loss seems to help with diabetes and diabetic risk factors but does not seem to help with stroke risk factors[170] (except for decreasing hypertension and its associated risks) – is this because after so many years the atherosclerosis has already been laid down and no amount of weight loss will get rid of it?

So duration and severity of obesity seem to limit the cardiovascular benefits of weight reduction in older men[171].

Regardless strive for at least 5-7% weight reduction in your at-risk patients anyway – it's our opinion that this can only help and not hurt. But the research clearly supports that it is far better to never have a weight problem and the sequelae that go along with that such as atherosclerosis.

5. Niaspan® (Nicotinic Acid)

Niacin as nicotinic acid broad-spectrum lipid drug, which lowers the concentration of all atherogenic plasma lipids while at the same time raising the levels of protective HDL[172], comes in three forms -- immediate-release (Niacor®), extended-release (Niaspan®), and slow-release (Endur-Acin®) and it is clear from the research that prescription niacin, such as niacin extended-release (Niaspan®), is efficacious and safe and should be the niacin product used to improve dyslipidemias[173]. Niaspan has considerable advantages over both immediate release and slow release (SR) formulations of this drug in that the major early side effect of immediate release niacin, the flush, is reduced with Niaspan[174].

Niaspan® Plus Crestor® For The Best Protection

Remember, lipoprotein(a), the major lipid risk factor for stroke atherogenesis, can only be reduced with niacin. We advise giving the ideal dose of 1000 mgm (1 gram) of Niaspan® every night (along with daily aspirin which reduces the flushing). Please inform your patients that after a week or so the flushing will pretty much cease. Niaspan® combines extremely well with rosuvastatin in stroke prevention and is a combination that should be your first choice with patients at risk[175].

6. B-Complex Vitamins and Folate To Reduce Homocysteine Levels

These B-complex and folate vitamins reduce homocysteine levels[176], sometimes dramatically, and can be taken by eating lots of green leafy vegetables but to make sure your patients are getting adequate amounts (always -- this is that critical) we advise a quality daily supplement (with a tablet containing a minimum of 2 mg of folate, 25 mg of B6, and 400 mcg of B12[177]).

7. Offset Sleep Apnea Risk Factors

Sleep apnea is associated with a 2-3 times increase in the normal risk for stroke. Though this relationship has only recently been strongly confirmed[178] it does seem at this time though the effects of treatment with continuous positive airway pressure (CPAP)[179] are very effective in at least partially reducing this risk. We strongly advise that if any of your patients have sleep apnea that you make every effort to reduce their cardiovascular and stroke risks as outlined in this chapter, regardless of whether they are on CPAP or not, including exercise and weight loss.

8. Offset Metabolic Syndrome Risk Factors

If you have metabolic syndrome patients or patients you suspect have metabolic syndrome treat them aggressively with a prescribed lifestyle modification program (exercise and diet/lifestyle changes) and aspirin, fish oil, alpha-lipoic acid (ALA), metformin, ezetimibe, rosuvastatin, and niacin at a minimum to reduce their risk for stroke. Please review Chapter 6 on type 2 diabetes prevention.

9. Control Lipids with a Statin

PROVE-IT-TIMI22

Lovastatin, a lipophilic compound, is able to cross the blood brain barrier and so would reasonably be the first choice for risk reduction in stroke but it increases lipoprotein(a) by over 20% making it not the first choice[180]. The PROVE-IT-TIMI-22 study showed that even with an LDL of 70 there was no reduction in risk but there was a dramatic reduction in risk in patients with lower (<2) CRP levels on atorvastatin (which does not cross the blood brain barrier)[181]. But the results of a large Chinese study indicated that atorvastatin protects against cerebral infarction via inhibition of NADPH oxidase-derived superoxide in transient focal ischemia[182].

CTT

In Austria, when there was a review of the Cholesterol Treatment Trialists' (CTT) Collaboration, the researchers came to the clear conclusion that a reduction in LDL-C using statins lead to a decrease in the incidence of strokes by 17%[183] and as a matter of fact each 10% reduction in LDL-cholesterol was estimated to reduce the risk of stroke by 15.6% in another large and excellent retrospective review[184]. Fatal strokes in this review were noted to be reduced by 9%. The Program 120® team believes that if rosuvastatin, which is the most potent statin and is lipophilic, was used in this study, it would have probably lowered LDL-C even further.

SPARCL

The Stroke Prevention by Aggressive Reduction in Cholesterol Levels[185] (SPARCL 2006) showed that high-dose statin therapy could significantly reduce the risk of stroke in individuals with a recent stroke but no evidence of coronary heart disease (CHD). SPARCL was the first randomized controlled clinical trial carried out to determine whether a daily statin dose would reduce the risk of stroke in patients who had suffered a stroke or transient ischemic attack (TIA) but had no known CHD (though they used atorvastatin at 80 mg in this study this shows you to push that dose of rosuvastatin to 40 mg if your prior stroke patients can tolerate it).

10. Quit Smoking and/or Drugs

Again, with future risk of strokes and the tiny microvasculature involved, the deleterious and long-lasting (sometimes a lifetime) effects of smoking, for even a short term, are horrendous – so it's much easier to say one should never start. And quitting decreases the risk of stroke as it does so many other diseases.

11. Lower hsCRP (Reduce Silent Inflammation) – Rosuvastatin Wins!

Highly sensitive C-reactive protein (hsCRP) is a biomarker for severe inflammation that has been highly predictive of stroke risk. There are a number of medications though that have been shown to reduce serum hsCRP levels: valsartan, rosuvastatin, pravastatin, lovastatin[186], and most significantly, atorvastatin[187]. Rosuvastatin, a lipophilic statin, seems to be the statin that's the most potent for the lowering of CRP[188].

But with this conclusion about rosuvastatin -- does it become the most potent anti-stroke statin? A recent Italian study involving stroke prone rats has shown that rosuvastatin is a potent anti-inflammatory neurovascular protectant[189].

The Program 120® team believes at this time the data clearly points to rosuvastatin as the best statin for preventing stroke, especially if started at a younger age.

12. Fish Oil

At Harvard a detailed study analysis indicated that any fish consumption conferred substantial relative stroke risk reduction compared to no fish consumption (12% for the linear model), and that additional consumption conferred incremental benefits (central estimate of 2.0% per serving per week)[190]. Extrapolation of this benefit could lead to as much as a 24% (or more) total decrease in stroke risk!

In the Division of Preventive Medicine at Brigham and Women's Hospital in a study among women who ate fish[191] it was shown among stroke subtypes, a significantly reduced risk of thrombotic infarction was found among women who ate fish 2 or more times per week, and for the women who ate the most fish, they had a 30% or greater reduction in thrombotic infarction. Fish consumption seemed to have no effect on hemorrhagic infarcts. We believe this research would be duplicated in men, also.

Certainly taking a potent fish oil capsule at least twice a day would gave the same benefits without the pollutions risk (mercury, PCBs, arsenic, etc). Remember, we believe that our patients should only be given "pharmaceutical grade" fish oil that has been "molecularly distilled" with as high DHA and EPA concentrations as possible (equivalent to 2,500 mgm a day of DHA + EPA).

.
Fish Oil Aids in the Treatment of Sickle Cell Thrombosis

At Grady Memorial Hospital in Georgia it was found that dietary n-3FAs (fish oil PUFAs) reduce the frequency of "pain episodes" by reducing prothrombotic activity in sickle cell disease and that this reduction was significant[192].

13. Aggressively Treat Atrial Fibrillation Risks

For a more thorough discussion of this subject we refer you to the landmark article by Singer DE, Albers GW, Dalen JE, Go AS, Halperin JL, Manning WJ – "Antithrombotic therapy in atrial fibrillation: the Seventh ACCP Conference on Antithrombotic and Thrombolytic Therapy." Published in Chest. 2004 Sep;126 (3 Suppl):429S-456S.

Low Risk: For patients with atrial fibrillation who are less than 65 years of age and carry no other risk factors, 325 mgm of aspirin a day (and not baby aspirins here) is sufficient[193].

Moderate Risk: In patients with persistent atrial fibrillation (AF) or paroxysmal atrial fibrillation (PAF), age 65 to 75 years, in the absence of other risk factors, the recommended antithrombotic therapy is with either an oral Vitamin K antagonists (VKA such as a warfarin or low-molecular weight heparinoid) or aspirin, 325 mg/d, in this group of patients who are at intermediate risk of stroke[194].

High Risk: In patients with persistent or PAF [intermittent AF] at high risk of stroke (i.e., having any of the following features: prior ischemic stroke, transient ischemic attack, or systemic embolism, age > 75 years, moderately or severely impaired left ventricular systolic function and/or congestive heart failure, history of hypertension, or diabetes mellitus), the recommended anticoagulation is with an oral VKA, such as warfarin[195].

For patients with AF and prosthetic heart valves, the recommended anticoagulation is with an oral VKA (Grade 1C+); the target INR may be increased and aspirin added depending on valve type and position, and on patient factors.

For patients with AF of ≥ 48 hours or of unknown duration for whom pharmacologic or electrical cardioversion is planned, the recommended anticoagulation is with an oral VKA for 3 weeks before and for at least 4 weeks after successful cardioversion (Grade 1C+ recommendation). For patients with AF of ≥48 h or of unknown duration undergoing pharmacologic or electrical cardioversion, an alternative strategy is anticoagulation and screening multiplane transesophageal echocardiography (Grade 1B). If no thrombus is seen and cardioversion is successful, the recommended anticoagulation is for at least 4 weeks (Grade 1B). For patients with AF of known duration <48 h, the suggestion is cardioversion without anticoagulation (Grade 2C). However, in patients without contraindications to anticoagulation, the suggestion is beginning IV heparin or low molecular weight heparin at presentation (Grade 2C)[196].

14. TZDs Shrink cIMT ➜ TZDs Prevent Strokes

When you get to Chapter 6, our chapter on diabetes, you will read more about thiazolidinediones (TZDs) or pioglitazone (Actos®) which, in our opinion, is the most effective thiazolidinedione because of its lipid actions – it primarily works by increasing/improving insulin sensitivity[197]. It is notable as to how well in concert it works with metformin[198] in preventing diabetes. **[BEWARE TZDs ALSO INCREASE THE RISK FOR BLADDER CANCER AS MENTIONED ELSEWHERE IN THIS MALE HEALTH BOOK – AUTHOR]**

But in stroke prevention and prevention of recurrence of an embolic or ischemic stroke it just might be king, especially in younger obese patients who already have a strong family history of stroke and type 2 diabetes. Pioglitazone, we know from the DREAM and PROActive[199] studies, appears to shrink atheroma size as measured by the cIMT

(Carotid Intimal Media Thickness) which is a huge significant prognostic indicator of stroke risk.

Read that again.

Rosiglitazone and pioglitazone shrink atheroma size as measured by the cIMT which is a huge significant prognostic indicator of stroke risk.

This the heart of the butterfly effect now spoken about by preventive medicine experts – start your patients young before they really even know they need it – you will add years to their lives. The interventional cardiologists now are asking why wait for these obese patient to develop full blown diabetes or to have a stroke while you primary care physicians debate on starting preventive maneuvers and medications. Start them now, today, on pioglitazone and they will reap HUGE benefits later.

Rosiglitazone and pioglitazone (from PROactive[200]) also improve free fatty acid (triglycerides) levels in the serum thus reducing insulin resistance through that mechanism, too[201].

Though minimal, this drug has its side effects. "Pioglitazone and rosiglitazone were associated with increased rates of hypoglycemia (17% and 11% of patients, respectively), significant weight gain (48% and 58%) and edema (33% and 21%).[202]"

Current Known Benefits of TZDs

1. PROActive Study results[203] showed improvement in a number of vascular areas reducing CHD risk dramatically (but these benefits occurred only with pioglitazone [Actos®]).
2. DREAM study[204] results show that using pioglitazone reduced the progression of metabolic syndrome patients to full diabetes by 60%.
3. TZDs prevent and reduce carotid atheromas (and cardiovascular atheroma) as measured by cIMT[205].
4. TZDs elevate HDL-C[206] (very hard to do!!!)
5. TZDs minimally lower LDL-C[207].
6. TZDs lower triglyceride dramatically[208].

7. TZDs act as Anti-Inflammatory meds aggressively reducing hsCRP[209].
8. TZDs lower coagulant levels in the blood reducing atherothrombotic risk[210].
9. TZDs act as vessel relaxants[211].
10. TZDs lower blood pressure (systolic and diastolic)[212].
11. TZDs elevate adiponectin[213]! Huh? This is cool! Adiponectin does so many good things that fight CHD.
12. TZDs, like ARBs, help prevent CKD (obviously by reducing diabetic factors), and they may be administered to treat diabetes in patients receiving hemodialysis, and they are considered safer than other oral hypoglycemic agents.
13. Thiazolidinediones also reduce insulin resistance, which is a risk factor for mortality in patients with ESRD[214].
14. Pioglitazone (Actos®) (and rosiglitazone) actually can shrink atheroma (measured by the cIMT) causing plaque regression[215].
15. Rosiglitazone and pioglitazone remove or regress fat deposits in muscles and other places – decreasing the inflammation there – a very important fact in diabetics and metabolic syndrome[216].
16. Rosiglitazone can completely remove or regress fat deposits in non-alcoholic steatohepatitis (NASH) or non-alcoholic fatty liver disease (NAFLD)[217], reducing the inflammation in the liver, also.
17. All this said there is the flip side -- pioglitazone (Actos®) has just been approved by the FDA for its lipid lowering effects[218] (lowers LDL and lipoprotein (a)) and we now believe this also has all the above benefits, too.
18. This cardiovascular protective effect has very recently been shown to not seem to be a class action effect but isolated to pioglitazone[219] (Actos®).

Need we say more? Start all of your at risk patients before they *really* need help, on pioglitazone at 15 mgm a day if you're nervous and it's just prevention. Push it to the maximum tolerated dose (45 mgm a day) while the patient is performing intensive lifestyle modification – save their lives now, not later after a stroke has occurred.

15. Proper Modern HRT

We refer you to our Chapter 11 on Modern Hormone Replacement Therapy. We advise you to conscientiously and aggressively treat your patient's menopausal and andropausal issues with modern biologically identical hormones. We think the literature is replete with articles that support this preventative step and have detailed them in the HRT section above and in Chapter 11. Stroke can and should be prevented and we, the members of the Program 120® team, believe that HRT is one of the most productive options for this prevention.

Acute Treatment of Stroke

Stroked? Reverse It ASAP! 3 Hours Max Limit!

Ischemic strokes are almost always amenable to "clot busting drugs" such as tissue plasminogen activator (tPA), the only U.S. Food and Drug Administration (FDA)-approved treatment for use in patients suffering from an acute ischemic stroke. Administered *within three hours* of the onset of symptoms, tPA can potentially break up the clot and possibly reduce disabilities caused by the stroke[220].

Whether the patient gets full recovery or not, especially in younger obese patients and ANY type 2 diabetic patients, that you make darn sure you have them on pioglitazone (Actos®) upon discharge as it is both neuroprotective and stroke preventing and from that day forward!

Quick Summary of Stroke Preventive Steps for Patients

1. BP should be 120/70
2. Use telmisartan (Micardis®) first to control
3. Quit smoking
4. Lose weight
5. Diet rich in vegetables and fruit
6. Control/unwind Metabolic Syndrome
7. Control/unwind type 2 diabetes – make sure these patients are on Actos®
8. No illicit drugs – they cause strokes
9. Control/unwind Sleep Apnea
10. Niaspan® 2000 mgm at night
11. Rosuvastatin or simvastatin at maximum dose (40 mgm)
12. Exercise at least 60 minutes every day (remember 1-4-7 FITT)
13. Lower hsCRP with B complex and folate

14. If at risk get a lipoprotein-associated phospholipase A(2) [Lp-PLA2]
15. Start HRT early as possible
16. Fish oil prevents, too (Res-Q-1250® 2-3X per day)
20. One half adult ASA every day
21. Treat hypothyroidism aggressively
22. Treat proteinuria aggressively with telmisartan (Micardis®)
23. Melatonin reduces risk – take at night to aid sleeping
24. Aggressively check for hypothyroidism and treat accordingly
25. TRT (testosterone) reduces stroke risk in hypogonadal men
26. Aggressively treat AF and PAF with ASA and VKA, etc.
27. Put all at risk patients (young and obese, type 2 diabetic, stroke family history, family history of type 2 diabetes and headed that way for sure) on at least 7.5 or 15 mgm of pioglitazone (Actos®) to prevent stroke. Save their lives. Do it before they really need help! You know who these patients are!
28. Remember, if you have a stroke get to a major hospital within 2-3 hours for
treatment and hopefully full recovery.

Chapter 27

I Have MS, am I Doomed?

No.

Top specialists and researchers (UCLA) actually say that testosterone levels should normalize in multiple sclerosis (MS) patients to prevent relapsing-remitting symptoms[221].

To the naysayers – I say why not? What does it hurt? If an MS patient had bronchitis, you'd treat them, right? If they had diabetes, you'd treat them, right? If the MS patient had a broken leg, you'd treat them, right?

Then why not treat MS patients with testosterone, since it can improve their demyelination[222] thus improving their MS.

We always treat if they wish it.

Chapter 28

I Have Male Fibromyalgia, am I Doomed?

First of all know, that I've written a book on fibromyalgia (Real Fibromyalgia Rx is available Amazon Kindle® or in paperback from Aesthetica PMI Press, LLC).

In 1990 Fibromyalgia Syndrome was given to the specialty of rheumatology to diagnose and treat – it's diagnosed by trigger points and other means. I don't think this matters as it should be under the purvey of endocrinologists (who are all already overworked and underpaid) who would probably scream if this occurred (if fibro was given to endocrinologists). It is given the term "syndrome," which essentially means what idiopathic means – no one knows the cause.

I call BS on that. The literature is clear on what causes fibromyalgia.

Fibromyalgia, in my opinion, is always from pituitary damage. And it's usually pretty severe damage. This level of damage almost always involves a growth hormone deficiency (called an AGHD or Adult Growth Hormone Deficiency).

We know from Italian studies[223] that statistically when you have even mild head trauma that human growth hormone (HGH) production is the most common thing affected negatively. Luteinizing hormone (LH) production is the second most commonly affected when the anterior pituitary is affected (so testosterone production is affected). FSH is next and then TSH is the least most affected of the anterior pituitary hormones. If you have all four affected (HGH, LH, FSH, and TSH), or at least three of them affected then you have the diagnosis of Panhypopituitarism.

And when no doctors can figure this out, you probably will then have the diagnosis of Fibromyalgia.

If this is the case, please get my book Real Fibromyalgia Rx which goes into the diagnosis and complex but proper therapy for this problem. You can, if treated properly and carefully, get rid of 95% of symptoms given enough time.

Chapter 29

I have Horrible Insomnia and Optimizing My Testosterone Did Not Help, Why Not?

First of all, insomnia sufferer, are you on any stimulants or caffeine or nicotine?

It always drives me CRAZY when patients complain about insomnia and then later admit to drinking a gallon of caffeine-laced soda (usually diet) or coffee, and smoking four (or twelve!!) packs of cigarettes a day.

Hello?

Those are stimulants!!! So please stop.

But I also practice in Utah where a significant number of my patients are Latter-day Saints (Mormon), who neither drink caffeinated beverages nor smoke.

Second of all I am pretty sure I've never seen a zolpidem deficiency!

I have, however, seen hypotestosteronism severely effect sleep and correcting or normalizing the testosterone deficiency can usually assist in somnolence and improving rest (sleep)[224].

So then it's back to the pituitary damage I've discussed throughout this book. The most common problem that occurs from pituitary damage is AGHD, or Adult Growth Hormone Deficiency. Lack of somatotropin (human growth hormone) causes severe insomnia or sleep disturbances[225] in most patients (think about a very poplar singer who recently passed away) along with severe fatigue symptoms. So these patients are exhausted all the time yet they cannot sleep or stay asleep. Lack of adequate growth hormone production leads to interruption in entering REM sleep (Rapid Eye Movement sleep – the lightest level of sleep) or staying asleep in Stage IV of sleep (deepest level of sleep).

These patients need to be worked up for an AGHD (or Adult Growth Hormone Deficiency) with proper stimulation testing (if available in your state). This is a complex disorder that requires proper evaluation. AGHD also leads to Sleep Apnea and is, in my opinion, the most common cause of this disorder (but yet it's never if ever mentioned to patients when they are diagnosed with sleep apnea).

Proper treatment with growth hormone and proper recovery/healing time allows patients to fall asleep normally (achieve normal REM) and to stay asleep (normal Stage IV).

Other than melatonin, I rarely (if ever) prescribe sleep aids or medications – it's back to my root cause belief system – deal with the root cause appropriately and then they will sleep more normally (some may require the addition of melatonin).

Know that melatonin works very well with growth hormone – there is a strong synergistic effect there that allows the melatonin to work. If you have a severe growth hormone deficiency, you may have tried melatonin before and thought it did not work – but try it after your AGHD has been properly dealt with and you'll usually see a huge difference in the way it works.

I start melatonin at a very low dose (300 mcg – that's MICROGRAMS) and increase the dose up until they sleep soundly for 6-8 hours. If they have a "hangover" or want to sleep in and watch the Price Is Right™ the next morning then their dose is too high – back it off a little.

My average patient dose is probably 5-10 mg (milligrams) a night of regular release (not timed release which I rarely suggest) melatonin.

Chapter 30

My Doctor Says You're Crazy, am I Doomed?

Give him this book and ask him to read it.

And if he does not?

Tell your doctor (uh oh) that he needs to read a study, or a book, or an article occasionally before he ignorantly spouts off about something of which he apparently knows not.

Then (again in my opinion), it might be time to find another physician who has some level of curiosity left in him or her. (The system can really beat it out of us physicians. My friend at USC who I do research with though is the MOST curious physician and researcher I have ever met and he was at Harvard, NIH and Walter Reed for 20 years *before* he was US Assistant Surgeon General, and he's not only a board certified endocrinologist but also a board certified cardiologist – he is the most credentialed physician in southern California but yet he's extremely curious. And yet other far less physicians think they already know it all? Truly unbelievable...)

Chapter 31

Male Contraception Options That Won't Hurt Me?

Ugh, touchy subject.

Getting your wife's/girlfriend's tubes tied is the best for most men but not always the best for women.

Condoms work really well and unless they're too small, they are definitely harmless.

Foams? They work too but make sure she applies it before you start.

Vasectomy is another option – but can be problematic if not done to exacting standards. I've seen several patients with pain down there for months or years later after vasectomy – and the exact reason remains unknown, but when we get their testosterone level back up pain occurs, probably in the area of the *vas deferens* so not always the best option in my book.

Injections of testosterone cypionate are also an option. Though far from fool proof, studies have shown that injection will usually prevent creation of any viable sperm[226].

Chapter 32

Will HCG give me "Man Boobs"? Aaargghh!
(And other potential side effects)

I get this question all the time – "βHCG is a female hormone – won't it give me man boobs?" (What you men is "gynecomastia".)

My answer is usually "You were smart enough to get in here (past my human wall, Mindi) to my practice, and now you're so ignorant as to ask that question? Really?"

And then I go onto say, "As I told you before I prescribed it, no, βHCG won't give you man or woman boobs, (or gynecomastia), because both sexes make it in the stalk of their pituitary."
And also remind them that the main concerns with βHCG are:

1. Infection at the site – so use lots of rubbing alcohol and clean it good before you give the shot!
2. And remember, though extremely rare, you could become allergic to βHCG, and then it won't work as well. This is like when patients become allergic to insulin and then they develop a resistance to the insulin. You will develop a resistance to the βHCG.

Not much in the way of side effects. Oh yes, and I have seen a couple of cases of borderline priapism.

If You Really Do Have Man "Boobs"?

This can happen if you take injectable tes cypionate (though actually I have never seen it with any of my thousands of patients). Then we ought to actually check an estradiol level and see where it falls. You actually might have high estradiol levels and we need to get you on an aromatase inhibitor (again, have never done this though).

Chapter 33

Stronger and Better Natural Erection Secrets?

It should be obvious to everyone that anything you do to increase or improve your overall circulation and health will improve your ability to attain better and stronger erections.

Exercise – Aerobic exercise improves cardiac output, cools blood vessels, reduces over all inflammation, and so improves circulation. When we did the research to write our textbook on preventive medicine[227], we looked at all the extensive research on exercise that Ralph Paffenbarger had done at Harvard with his "Harvard Professional" studies ("College Alumni Health Study" as it was more formally known), we concluded that when you "smashed" all his data and various studies together you get what we termed "1-4-7."

1-4-7 means just to *maintain* weight and cardiovascular health, the average human should do 1 hour of exercise a day, and it should be done on an equivalent to walking 4 miles per hour (a *brisk* walk according to Paffenbarger), and it should be done, if possible, 7 days a week – thus the 1-4-7.

And that's what we advise people to do just to *maintain* weight and fitness. We chose walking because most people can easily walk somewhere every day. What we find people have the most difficulty with was the time of 1 hour – in today's rushed world few people has that much time to work out. But, according to Paffenbarger's excellent data, that's the minimum you should do every day.

If you wish to improve your fitness (especially for the bedroom) you need to do a little more than walking 4 miles per hour (such as work up to 5 miles per hour, but do it slowly and only after physician approval) *plus* cut back on your calories (just a little). Amazing things will most likely happen.

Especially in the bedroom.

(Got it? Your goal might or should be 1 hour of walking at 5 miles per hour, plus cut back on your calories. Harder than it sounds but not impossible.)

Weight Loss – If you do what I just suggested, the weight loss will come. Our only rule is to weigh daily, at the same time, on the same scales. Watch things closely.

Lower that High Blood Pressure – Lowering high blood pressure properly has been shown in a number of studies to help with improving ED[228], plus obviously adding stamina and endurance in bed. But what we just said is deeper and more complex than it sounds because we used the word "properly."

How do you properly lower high blood pressure? For years doctors lowered blood pressure however they could – what the cuff said was the proof. Then a group of physicians doing a really large research study[229] discovered that some patients, who appeared to have properly controlled blood pressure, were still dying at a rate and from diseases of untreated hypertension. Curious, they decided to check central or aortic blood pressures and found that *they were essentially uncontrolled.* They then concluded that some blood pressure meds would lower blood pressure in the peripheral blood vessels but *not centrally* where it counts. So they then concluded the following method of stepwise blood pressure medicine prescription was what worked:

1. The goal is to get blood pressure down to below 120/70. At below 120/70 patients tend to get plaque regression. You want this – it's a good thing, because that means plaque leaves your arteries (especially arteries *in your penis*) helping maintain your life *and* your love life.
2. Start on an ACE Inhibitor (such as cheap generic lisinopril) as the first line. This works centrally as do all the following meds. If the ACE inhibitor does not work, add the mild diuretic, HCTZ (hydrochlorothiazide). It now helps that a lot of blood pressure meds, even generics, come combined with HCTZ.
3. If these two do not do it, add the medication amlodipine, which is a is a long-acting calcium channel blocker, acts by relaxing the smooth muscle in the arterial wall, decreasing total peripheral resistance and hence reducing blood pressure; in angina, it increases blood flow to the heart muscle. So it only goes to believe that amlodipine will also increase blood flow to your penis and the arteries there to help cause and maintain an erection.
4. You need to max out each medicine at each step before you move on to the next level.
5. If in the end (I've never seen this but am sure it can occur) all this just does not work (in normalizing the blood pressure), you can also try medicine variants within each category – for example nifedipine as the calcium channel blocker instead of amlodipine.

And remember all these meds have many potential side effects, so it's actually much simpler and less problematic to lose weight and increase exercise in order to bring down your blood pressure, but make sure it's under control while you do it.

Adequate L-arginine -- such as you'd fine in the excellent MLM supplement Pro-Argi-9+™ by Synergy® or Pro-Arginine Plus® (available on Amazon) which you should take as directed. There has been all kind of studies that show this improved NO, or Nitric Oxide, which can improve circulation and vascular dilatation. NO has been shown to directly cause increased blood flow to the penis. And L-arginine, in adequate amounts daily, can improve NO production[230].

Glutathione – Glutathione, in its reduced form (called GSH), can increase NO production, which in turn (see above) increases blood flow to the penis for better erections. Reduced glutathione (GSH) historically is incredibly unstable (it reacts even with the oxygen in air, it's that aggressive an anti-oxidant), and short-lived. Here are some things that can help with production:

1. **NAC** or N-acetyl cysteine taken daily can help with production of GSH. NAC is the rate limiting amino acid in the production of the tripeptide, glutathione (see the book I wrote on glutathione). If you don't have enough NAC none of this other stuff matters.

2. **Topical Lime or Orange oil** (I prefer Young Living Essential Oils™), at 8 drops a day, smells really good and can increase your own internal glutathione production, actually pretty dramatically. We know it does this because I've checked blood levels myself of before and after but more importantly, it contains tons of citrol and d-limonene which have been shown to increase GSH production.

3. **RealGSH™** is a topical and cosmetic stable and complexed glutathione spray that my team and I developed and have a patent pending on. It's really just a super blast of anti-oxidant goodness which

can really help your glutathione levels. No promises or claims here, but it might be worth a try. Find the website (www.realgsh.com) and use code DRPTESBOOK to get a 10% discount.

4. Note if you take or increase your glutathione levels you need to increase your CoQ10 levels too. Take lots of CoQ10, especially if you have a busy sex life.

Cialis™ or Viagra™ or Levitra™ -- I guess this subject matter and chapter would be incomplete if I did not add a section on these medications. They have a viable place in this discussion but only as secondary or tertiary options after hormone levels, exercise, weight loss, and blood pressure concerns are all properly and thoroughly addressed. The main idea of these medications, from a therapeutic direction, are to improve circulation by inhibiting cGMP-specific phosphodiesterase type 5, an enzyme that promotes degradation of cGMP, which regulates blood flow in the penis, allowing increased blood flow to enter the penis and to stay there, causing an erection or an improved erection.

Chapter 34

Are Male Multiple Orgasms Possible?

In a word, yes, some rare men can have more orgasms in one sex session. But I think if you need to read this book, having multiple orgasms is probably not even a consideration – you're probably more worried about just getting an erection and having the rare orgasm.

But some of you might be concerned and curious about this and so you know it is possible. You better be very fit and loaded with vitamins and amino acids – because you'll need them.

There are websites dedicated to this proposal:

http://multiplemaleorgasm.org/

http://www.pegym.com/articles/the-multiple-male-orgasm

Beyond this – this topic is probably outside the scope of this text.

Chapter 35

Improving Sexuality and Sperm Viability – a Summary

Producing more viable sperm is really what this book was originally intended to do – it's something many of my patients desire and really need help with.

Hopefully I have listed the minefields that can destroy your sperm and the help meets that can improve your chances of getting your loved one pregnant.

Let's review them one more time – first let's go through the list of

Things you can do:

Exercise
Lose Weight – get to a normal weight
Lift Weights
Take adequate amino acids
Get a SpectraCell™ -- get your vitamins right!
Take lots of L-arginine and fish oil, too!
Take lots of CoQ10 (even if your levels are normal on SpectraCell™)
Get your testosterone levels checked
If needed, only use βHCG as therapy for low tes
If it's Primary Hypogonadism use a cream or tes injectable.

Things to avoid:

Cell phone in your pocket
Laptop on your lap
Laziness
A pot belly
Low tes levels
Tes cypionate (unless it's your only option that works)
Radiation
Infections

Chapter 36

Frequently Asked Questions (And Answers)

Will normalizing my tes levels cause me to go bald?

A genetic condition called Male Pattern Baldness causes you to go bald, not actually testosterone. Of interest though, a breakdown byproduct of testosterone, dihydroepitestosterone (DHT), attacking the hair root is the hormonal cause of hair loss so indirectly the answer may be yes, BUT your tes levels would have to near zero for this condition to not kick in and then you'd just die, with a full head of hair probably (lying in your casket) but you'd be dead.

If this is a concern I refer you to the website

http://www.thebaldtruth.com

which is excellent and full of information. But my overriding belief is to be healthy and virile and bald – you can use Rogaine™ while you're dating, but at least you'll be alive and dating.

Shouldn't I be on an Aromatase Inhibitor for the estradiol?

This is one of those questions that make me wonder, "Where doe this stuff come from?"

The next thing I ask myself is should I have put the young man who had a natural tes level of 1432 ng/dl on an aromatase inhibitor then?

My answer to all this is no. Here's why:

The theory behind this question is high testosterone levels will be aromatized (converted) to the female hormone estradiol. And that will give you feminizing characteristics. There are a few problems with theory.

First problem or fact is that if men have extra testosterone (very rare but let's go there for the sake of discussion) they do convert some to estradiol but this has been determined to be done in the body for the estradiol's cardio-protective benefits (estradiol in men increases flexibility of the arteries while aromatase inhibitors increase arterial stiffness[231] when they lower estradiol). So in actuality it's a good thing. It's also important to point out at this point that men always have a little estradiol in them.

Second problem (or fact) is that no one's really determined at what level is the level of estradiol "high" and what bad things happen when it's high. So I ask my patients who request this estradiol level, "Well what level will we consider too high?"

And they can never answer me. NO ONE KNOWS.

So there is NOT an answer. And for this you want a $300 a month aromatase inhibitor? (I'll prescribe it if you really want, but it's waste of money.)

There is also an opposing opinion out there – and it is viable and well thought through. This is why include the recent excellent work being done out there on how to reboot the hypothalamus (see Chapter 12 and the associated references).

What is my estradiol level?

Same.

Is my estradiol level too high?

Only if you want an aromatase inhibitor

Won't that excess tes convert to estradiol and give me "man boobs"?

No. Those are more than likely your pecs coming back – try to lift some weights.

My back is breaking out ("backne") so I am stopping everything, is that okay?

No. Instead let's just reduce your tes levels a little and back way off on the DHEA also we can add a little oral or topical doxycycline.

I feel really good now but all these hormones are causing me to gain weight, so I am stopping them, is that okay?

Did you come to me for weight loss or to get better and feel better? And which is more important – your weight or your health? My advice would also be to avoid carbs and eat more protein, too. Start working out more too.

Doesn't the HCG work better if I give it IM?

Some studies have suggested that but take it however you want, but please JUST TAKE IT (my biggest concern).

Doesn't the HCG work better if I give it deep IM with a really long needle?

I guess if you enjoy the pain. Again some studies and historical evidence tend to support the theory that deep IM HCG works better but take it however you want, just take it.

Why did my leg swell up and turn red where I gave my tes shot?

You may have hit a vein or lacerated a tiny artery – so use some warm moist heat on the area and don't give more shots that area any time soon. I also see this when patients don't scrub the area with alcohol really good before giving a shot. If this is the case, then watch for other signs of infection and let's get you on an antibiotic.

My primary care doc now says my tes levels have become normal so I don't need these meds any more -- so I'm stopping everything, is that okay?

Huh? Think about what you're saying here and reason with me – you're tes levels are now normal because you're taking all of this. Trust me, you have not magically been cured. I am good, but I'm certainly not God. Take your meds and stay on track.

And definitely find a new and more intelligent primary care doctor.

My libido is not as good as I thought it would be, so why take all this?

Did you come to me just for your libido or everything else and maybe your libido? Libido is so hard to return to "normal" (really hard in women) and you're broken – you will never be perfect again nor will everything (including your libido) be optimal again – again, YOU'RE BROKEN!

And medicine, as good as it is, is not that good. At best, this is just a poor imitation of how Heavenly Father (i.e. God or Allah or your Higher Power) designed us to work.

This stuff is expensive, is there anything cheaper?

No. I am always shopping for the cheapest and most natural options for my patients. Don't come to me if you can't live with my recommendations, please -- it is a waste of my time and your money.

This stuff is too expensive and my buddy at the gym says he can get it for me a LOT cheaper, is this okay?

Good luck with that. And don't do it. And if you do, don't come back to me.

My testicles have shrunk, huh?

Remember my "poor imitation" comment (see above)? Well, injectable or cream testosterone tends to cause the testicles to shrink because it suppresses their function. But on the other hand, it tends to make the penis longer and thicker, so it's a trade off. Taking injectable HCG will prevent this though.

I'm really horny now, so can I give my wife a shot of this tes cypionate every once in a while to help her?

First of all, testosterone in any form is a controlled substance and using it any way beyond how it was prescribed is illegal, so don't do this. Also, injectable or men's topical tes cream or gel is at an excessively high concentration which for females is not safe. Too high of tes levels in women makes them *very* angry – so good luck with that.

I'm really horny now, so can I give my wife a touch of this tes cream/gel every once in a while to help her?

Same as the shot. No, it's too high a concentration.

I'm really horny now, so what can I give my wife to help her?

Try flowers. If that doesn't work then do the dishes.

If all that doesn't work, then have her come and see me – I actually deal with more women than men.

I'm single and celibate so I don't want to have ANY libido so I am quitting all this stuff, is that okay?

It's not okay with me but do whatever you want. Sorry you can't control your own thoughts and libido – how many guys though would be jealous of your position? But it's a free country (still, kinda) so you can do whatever you want.

My VAH doctor says testosterone is "cosmetic" so what do you say?

After a bitter laugh I usually say this approach, by calling a problem a "non-problem (huh?), is absurd. This is a bunch of ignorant bureaucrats making a cost saving decision. This book and my textbook clearly explains what I believe.

My insurance company won't pay for this so is this stuff, so is it all bogus?

You need to choose who to believe. Insurance companies hire a bunch of nurse (LPNs and some RNs) to review billings. Then these nurses can go to some retired elderly physician, hired as a medical director who knows little to nothing about this area, for any final decisions. My past observations is that these medical directors are then advised by a team of "handlers" who are just insurance company hacks. They almost all know next to nothing and are usually vile and nasty people who could not care less about your health or the medical literature and what it says.

So you're letting them make your medical decisions for you?

You probably came to the wrong physician.

Can I reuse the needles?

Sure if you want an infection. Or you live in a crack house. So no.

I refrigerated my tes cypionate, and now it has crystals in it -- can I still use it?

No, it's ruined.

My HCG has turned cloudy or brown/green/purple/red/black, is it safe to use?

No, it's ruined.

Won't injecting this tes protect me from STDs?

No it will not. Condoms will or staying celibate will.

My friend/mom/doc gave me an article from 1957 that says tes cypionate will kill me -- what say you?

(You'd be surprised how often I get this.) Dig back deep enough and you can find articles showing that smoking cigarettes will improve your health. So please don't waste my time.

I'm taking all these natural supplements for my tes, and they work -- why didn't you mention them?

Clearly I am not as knowledgeable as you – please write a book and tell us more. And this book is limited to my knowledge which is very finite.

Is it true if you eat a raw bull's testicle every week, that you don't need all this stuff?

If true I say "Wow, really? Then you don't need me or my years of education, training, and practice experience. Eat up, cowboy!"

Can I ask you REALLY personal questions on Facebook?

Yes, but people may laugh or reel back in shocked horror and doubtful I will answer because HIPAA privacy laws are brutal.

Can I ask you 3 paragraph long free medical questions on Facebook?

Yes, but I probably won't answer it. I am not a surgeon I am a cognitive physician –- C-O-G-N-I-T-I-V-E -- so I don't get paid for procedures but for my thinking skills and brain work (knowledge). I don't mind answering a brief question (I have 5,000+ friends on Facebook as this written so you can imagine how bad this can be) but why should I give my skills away to a complete stranger or to anyone on the internet? That's like one of my partners/associates performing free surgery on the highway, or in an airport or library, or like Wal-Mart™ giving away free groceries – doesn't happen (though I often see less

143

advantaged and needy patients for free – I'll even pay for their care and labs and meds – but I choose these).

I want you to call and talk to my doctor/insurance company/wife/girl friend, when can I set that up?

This does not sound fun or helpful. To anyone. I will do it but please understand that all these calls and requests (you're not the only one) are a HUGE time suck and add stress to my day, so please offer to reimburse me for my time.

Why won't you bill my insurance for me and just accept what they pay?

Hahahahahahahah! Are you kidding? First of all, they'd tell me and you how you can be treated! Really? Some review nurse or some old crusty retired doctor telling us how to treat you? No thanks.

I'd also have to hire all new staff to deal with these "companies." And I'd have to sign up with various plans and that means signing contracts that no sane person or intelligent business person would EVER sign. Then the insurance companies can "investigate" me or argue with me or deny and recover monies from me even when I've seen you and given you care. That's piracy or thievery in most countries of the world. So we're not going there. I will quit practicing first before I ever do that.

Refer to http://www.aaps.org

for my position on this matter.

I actually wish that there were NO third party payers to intercede in your care. That's how extreme I am.

My insurance company doesn't believe you, will you call and talk to them?

See the two answers I just gave above.

My insurance company wants you to get "pre-authorization" for this HCG or tes cypionate that YOU ordered, why haven't you called them?

It's not my job. It's not part of my duties – I did not sign up with them – you did. Regardless, my agreement is between you and I regarding your care. Also, what happens if they say no?

So please, you call them.

Will you coordinate your care of me with my family doctor?

Sure, I'll send him/her a nice letter, but trust me he does not have an hour or even 5 minutes to chat with me. A letter will suffice. IF he calls though of course I will talk to him. No problem.

My doc won't order these labs you suggest, so how do I get them?

That's certainly their choice and right. Either live with it or find another doc or go to my website:

http://www.danpursermd.com

There you can find a way to get your labs (and NO, insurance will NOT pay for them and NO we will not give you a diagnostic code, and NO we will not give you away to bill your insurance) -- this is strictly a cash or credit card only option but we've tried to set prices accordingly PLUS you can get them drawn pretty much anywhere in the USA (big city only though), so it's a good last resort option.

A note from Dr. Purser

If you enjoyed this book and found it helpful please feel free to leave a review on Amazon on my Kindle book page (under the book title). It is MUCH appreciated and puts you in the running to win other free books with contests we occasionally have (in the future).

If you wish to order this book in paperback please go to my website and order it there:

www.danpursermd.com

Also, if your physician won't or can't (as is often the case nowadays) order you the specific labs you request (which I suggest in this book) – on the above website you will also see a button for Direct Labs – just click on that and follow their directions. It is a cheap and easy way to get labs locally near you and to pay cash (actually a credit card I believe) – just know that insurance will not cover these nor can you get reimbursed as no diagnostic code will be issued (how can we? We don't even know you nor have we seen you…).

Thanks so much for purchasing AND reading this book – your seeking for knowledge in a confusing world is much appreciated.

--Dan Purser, MD

Important Web Pages

My Web Pages: ☺

My practice website:

http://www.aespmi.com

My Dan Purser MD info web page:

http://www.danpursermd.com

My Amazon Author Page

http://www.amazon.com/s/ref=ntt_athr_dp_sr_1?_encoding=U TF8&field-author=Dan%20Purser&search-alias=digital-text&sort=relevancerank

My Facebook Page (or search for Dan Purser MD and like me)

https://www.facebook.com/pages/Dan-Purser-MD/352156728226618

(If you wish to communicate with me, please "LIKE ME"!!!)

Freedom in medical practice web page (The Association of American Physicians and Surgeons):

http://www.aaps.org

Best hair loss web page:

http://www.thebaldtruth.com

Male multiple orgasm pages:

http://multiplemaleorgasm.org/

http://www.pegym.com/articles/the-multiple-male-orgasm

MLM Web Pages (for which I consult):

Young Living's Essential Oil Web Page (official)

NuSkin's Web Page

The RealGSH (glutathione) Web Page

http://www.realgsh.com

(Try some!!!)

Best Compounding Pharmacy Web Pages (for compounded HCG or Tes Cream or Gel):

Central Drugs in La Habra, California (these guys are the BEST in California and are a bunch of PharmDs who teach at USC:

http://centraldrugsrx.com/

MedQuest in Utah (they are excellent and can ship ANYWHERE in the world):

http://www.mqrx.com

The MedQuest educational website – for educating physicians in regards to hormones and how to properly prescribe them.

http://www.worldlinkmedical.com/

AWESOME Doctor's Websites:

Jeffrey Dach, MD in Florida (the man to see in Florida – does great work and great blog):

http://www.drdach.com/home.html

Neal Rouzier, DO in California who is a thought leader in this field.   http://hormonedoctor.com

INDEX

ADHD, 23, 61

allicin, 64

amino acid deficiency, 32, 43, 65, 81

amyotrophic lateral sclerosis

    ALS, Lou Gehrig's Disease, 38

anterior pituitary dysfunction, 30, 40

Australia, 103

Azoospermia

    azoospermia. See sperm

benign erythrocytosis, 14, 20

bipolar disorder, 23, 59

blood pressure, 10, 11, 13, 24, 30, 37, 88, 91, 98, 104, 105, 106, 107, 108, 115, 129, 130, 132

brush border, 23

CBC

    Complete Blood Count, 14, 20

Central Drugs. See compounding pharmacy

Central Hypogonadism. See pituitary hypogonadism, Pituitary, Hypogonadotrophic Hypogonadism, See pituitary hypogonadism, Pituitary, Hypogonadotrophic Hypogonadism, See pituitary hypogonadism, Pituitary, Hypogonadotrophic Hypogonadism, See pituitary hypogonadism, Pituitary, Hypogonadotrophic Hypogonadism, See pituitary hypogonadism, Pituitary, Hypogonadotrophic Hypogonadism

cholesterol, 10, 21, 56, 64, 88, 98, 104, 110

Cialis™

    phosphodiesterase inhibitor. See phosphodiesterase inhibitor, See phosphodiesterase inhibitor

Clomid™

    clomiphene citrate. See hypothalamus reboot, See hypothalamus reboot, See hypothalamus reboot, See hypothalamus reboot, See hypothalamus reboot

cognitive, 91, 144

concussion

    concussive, 37, 59, 60

constipation, 23

CoQ10

    CoEnzyme Q10, 20, 44, 45, 56, 57, 63, 83, 84, 99, 132, 134

cortisol

    Cortisol, 13, 19, 39

cream, 32, 33, 34, 56, 66, 70, 71, 77, 134

Cytomel™

    FT3, L-thyronine. See FT3, L-thyronine

damaged pituitary, 17, 60

DEA, 32, 80

depression, 15, 23, 44, 48, 52, 60, 93, 97, 98, 104

DHA

    Fish Oil. See Fish Oil, See Fish Oil, See Fish Oil, See Fish Oil, See Fish Oil, See Fish Oil, See Fish Oil, See Fish Oil, See Fish Oil, See Fish Oil, See Fish Oil, See Fish Oil, See Fish Oil, See Fish Oil, See Fish Oil, See Fish Oil

DHEA

    DeHydroEpiAndrosterone, 12, 17, 19, 44, 155

dihydroepitestosterone

    DHT. See Male Pattern Baldness

doxycycline

    backne. See

dry ejaculation, 18

EPA. See DHA, Fish Oil, fish oil, See DHA, Fish Oil, fish oil, See DHA, Fish Oil, fish oil, See DHA, Fish Oil, fish oil, See DHA, Fish Oil, fish oil, See DHA, Fish Oil, fish oil, See DHA, Fish Oil, fish oil, See DHA, Fish Oil, fish oil, See DHA, Fish Oil, fish oil, See DHA, Fish Oil, fish oil, See

DHA, Fish Oil, fish oil, See DHA, Fish Oil, fish oil
erectile dysfunction
ED, Erectile Dysfunction, 15, 20, 89, 90, 98, 104
FDA, 30, 32, 48, 53, 55, 56, 67, 75, 82, 115, 116
fibromyalgia
male fibromyalgia. See anterior pituitary dysfunction, RealFibromyalgiaRx, See anterior pituitary dysfunction, RealFibromyalgiaRx
fluoxetine
Prozac. See depression, See depression
food allergy, 23
football
NFL, concussion, 29, 37, 59, 70
Free Testosterone
free testosterone, 11, 103
FT3
L-thyronine, Free T3, 12, 20, 39, 56
German chamomile. See YLEO, See YLEO, See YLEO
Glutathione
glutathione. See RealGSH, www.realgsh.com, See RealGSH, www.realgsh.com, See RealGSH, www.realgsh.com, See RealGSH, www.realgsh.com, See RealGSH, www.realgsh.com
gluten intolerance, 23
HbA1C. See diabetes, diabetics
HCG, 7, 17, 54, 56, 68, 126, 139, 141, 143, 146, 150
head blows, 29
headaches
migraine, 10, 15, 22
heart attack
MI, 14, 20, 21, 39, 58, 97, 99
HGH, 90, See
HIPAA

privacy laws, 144
hsCRP
highly sensitive C-Reactive Protein, 14, 21, 22, 111, 115, 117
hyperthyroidism, 20
hypothalamus, 32, 41
hypothalamus reboot. See Clomid, See Clomid, See Clomid, See Clomid, See Clomid
hypothyroidism
FT3, 38, 40, 104, 117
IGF-1
Insulin Like Growth Factor 1, 12, 18, 19, 99
Imetrex®. See migraine headaches
injectable testosterone. See cypionate, enanthate, propionate, See cypionate, enanthate, propionate, See cypionate, enanthate, propionate, See cypionate, enanthate, propionate
insomnia. See AGHD, HGH, See AGHD, HGH, See AGHD, HGH, See AGHD, HGH
Jeffrey Dach, MD, 150
kidney
BUN, Creatinine, creatinine, 14, 22
Laminine™. See amino acid deficiency, Amina Acid Deficiency, See amino acid deficiency, Amina Acid Deficiency, See amino acid deficiency, Amina Acid Deficiency
L-arginine, 43, 46, 58, 131, 134
L-Carnitine
seminiferous tubules, 46
Levitra™
phosphodiesterase inhibitor. See phosphodiesterase inhibitor
Lexapro™, 10
Leydig cell, 96
LH, 11, 17, 18, 19, 29, 30, 31, 38, 41, 52, 53, 55, 65, 66, 75, 119, 155
LHRH. See hypothalamus

151

luteinizing hormone releasing hormone, 31
libido, 9, 10, 11, 12, 13, 15, 19, 20, 31, 32, 34, 36, 38, 41, 42, 44, 45, 52, 60, 63, 64, 67, 86, 89, 90, 98, 155
liver enzymes
ALT, AST, 14
L-ornithine, 46
low testosterone, 10, 11, 15, 17, 25, 29, 41, 53, 59, 60, 61, 70, 87, 93, 102, 103
Male Pattern Baldness
bald. See
Man-opause
Manopause, manopause, 6, 36
Mayo Clinic, 78, 90
MedQuest, 45, 77, 150, See
compounding pharmacy
MedQuest®
World's Largest Compounding Pharmacy, 77
melatonin. See insomnia, See insomnia, See insomnia, See insomnia, See insomnia, See insomnia
Migraine headaches
Migraine, migraines, migraine, cluster, 101
MILD HYPOGONADISM
mild hypogonadism, 26
mineral deficiency, 43
MLB®, 30
Multiple Sclerosis
MS, 23, 91
multiplemaleorgasm, 133, 149
NAC
Cysteine, cysteine. See glutathione, See glutathione, See glutathione, See glutathione, See glutathione
NCAA®, 30
Neal Rouzier, DO, 150
nicotinic acid
Niaspan, niacin. See
Novarel™

βHCG. See βHCG, Human Chorionic Gonadotropin, Cialis
NUMBER 1 CAUSE
#1, 29
Nuvigil™, 10
obesity, 13, 73, 103, 105, 108
Omega-3 Ultra Potency Fish Oil™
fish oil. See DHA, EPA, Oleic Acid
pituitary tumor, 30
Plaque regression
plaque regression. See heart attack, stroke
polycythemia vera, 14, 91
Polyglandular Autoimmune Type II Syndrome
Polyglandular Autoimmune Type II Syndrome, 13
pot
marijuana, 62, 70, 74, 135
Pregnenolone
pregnenolone, 44
Pregnyl™. See βHCG, Novarel
priapism, 126
primary hypogonadism
central hypogonadism, pituitary hypogonadism, hypogonadotrophic hypogonadism, 16
propionate, 34, 79, 80
prostate cancer. See PSA, See PSA, See PSA, See PSA, See PSA, See PSA, See PSA, See PSA, See PSA, See PSA, See PSA, See PSA, See PSA, See PSA, See PSA, See PSA, See PSA, See PSA
Provigil™, 10
PSA
Prostate Specific Antigen, 7, 13, 20, 87, 92, 155
Qunol™
CoQ10. See CoQ10, ubiquinol, See CoQ10, ubiquinol, See CoQ10, ubiquinol
radiation. See , See , See
RealFibromyalgiaRx
Kindle, Amazon, 119

rosuvastatin
Crestor. See plaque regression,
See plaque regression, See
plaque regression, See plaque
regression, See plaque
regression, See plaque
regression, See plaque
regression, See plaque
regression, See plaque
regression
Selenium
selenium. See hypothyroidism,
See hypothyroidism
Sertoli cell, 96
SEVERE HYPOGONADISM
severe hypgonadism, 26
SHBG
Sex Hormone Binding Globulin,
11, 12, 79, 88
shrink. See testicles, See testicles,
See testicles, See testicles
Simvastatin. See plaque regression,
See plaque regression, See plaque
regression, See plaque regression
Sloan Kettering Institute, 68
SpectraCell® Comprehensive
Micronutrient Analysis Panel. See
SpectraCell®
Spectracell™. See Vitamin, Amino
Acide Deficiency, Mineral
Deficiency
sperm, 11, 18, 31, 32, 34, 38, 41, 43,
44, 45, 46, 47, 52, 53, 56, 63, 64,
65, 66, 67, 70, 71, 72, 73, 74, 81,
82, 95, 125, 134
spermatogenesis, 46, 47, 90
stalk, 30, 126
stroke
CVA, 14, 20, 21, 30, 39, 58, 82, 97,
102, 103, 104, 105, 106, 108,
109, 110, 111, 112, 113, 114,
115, 116, 117
telmisartan
Micardis®, Priotor®). See , See ,
See , See , See , See
temperature, 71, 72

testicular cancer, 31, 74, 95, 96
testicular cancer, seminoma, 95
testosterone cypionate, 34, 56, 71,
79, 125
testosterone enanthate, 16, 80
Tobacco
smoking, 73
total testosterone, 11, 15, 16, 55, 88,
89
Total Testosterone
total testosterone, TT, 11, 15, 17,
25, 26, 56, 87
transferrance, 33, 77, 78
trauma, 13, 29, 30, 32, 36, 37, 38, 42,
59, 60, 66, 70, 74, 104, 119
Traumatic Brain Injury
TBI, 37
triglycerides. See MI, CVA, stroke,
heart attack, See MI, CVA, stroke,
heart attack, See MI, CVA, stroke,
heart attack
ubiquinol
Qunol, CoQ10. See CoQ10, See
CoQ10, See CoQ10
US Assistant Surgeon General
board certified pituitary
endocrinologist, 124
Vagal Nerve demyelination, 23
varicocele, 73
vascular inflammation
hsCRP, 14, 21, 22, 24, 81, 98, 102
vascular stiffness, 24, 103
Viagra™
phosphodiesterase inhibitor. See
Cialis, See Cialis, See Cialis
vitamin, 17, 32, 42, 43, 45, 47, 48, 50,
53, 64, 65, 67
www.drsinatra.com
Stephen Sinatra, MD. See CoQ10
Yoga
yoga, stretching, 86
Young Living Essential Oils™
YLEO. See German chamomile,
Omegagize3
zinc
Zinc, 43, 47, 63

153

[1] Gleicher N, Barad DH. Dehydroepiandrosterone (DHEA) supplementation in diminished ovarian reserve (DOR). Reprod Biol Endocrinol. 2011 May 17;9:67. doi: 10.1186/1477-7827-9-67.

[2] Bloch M, Meiboom H, et al. The use of dehydroepiandrosterone in the treatment of hypoactive sexual desire disorder: A report of gender differences. Eur Neuropsychopharmacol. 2012 Oct 17. pii: S0924-977X(12)00268-4. doi: 10.1016/j.euroneuro.2012.09.004.

[3] Accessed online 15 February 2013. http://en.wikipedia.org/wiki/Androstenedione#cite_note-ReferenceA-4.

[4] Broeder, CE; Quindry, J; Brittingham, K; Panton, L; Thomson, J; Appakondu, S; Breuel, K; Byrd, R et al. (2000). "The Andro Project: Physiological and hormonal influences of androstenedione supplementation in men 35 to 65 years old participating in a high-intensity resistance training program". Archives of Internal Medicine 160 (20): 3093–3104.

[5] Mendivil Dacal JM, Borges VM. [Dehydroepiandrosterone (DHEA), review of its efficiency in the managing of the libido decrease and other symptoms of aging]. [Article in Spanish] Actas Urol Esp. 2009 Apr;33(4):390-401.

[6] Savineau JP, Marthan R, et al. Role of DHEA in cardiovascular diseases. Biochem Pharmacol. 2012 Dec 25. pii: S0006-2952(12)00790-3. doi: 10.1016/j.bcp.2012.12.004.

[7] Ogura T, Mimura Y, et al. Hypothyroidism associated with anti-human chorionic gonadotropin antibodies secondarily produced by gonadotropin therapy in a case of idiopathic hypothalamic hypogonadism. J Endocrinol Invest. 2003 Nov;26(11):1128-35.

[8] Gold PW, Kling MA, et al. Corticotropin releasing hormone: relevance to normal physiology and to the pathophysiology and differential diagnosis of hypercortisolism and adrenal insufficiency. Adv Biochem Psychopharmacol. 1987;43:183-200.

[9] Das SK, Ghosh A, et al. A patient with recurrent attacks of drowsiness and lethargy--a diagnosis not to be missed. J Indian Med Assoc. 2012 May;110(5):327, 329.

[10] Raynaud JP, Gardette J, et al. Prostate-specific antigen (PSA) concentrations in hypogonadal men during 6 years of transdermal testosteronetreatment. BJU Int. 2013 Jan 7. doi: 10.1111/j.1464-410X.2012.11514.

[11] Caminos-Torres R, Ma L, Snyder PJ. Testosterone-induced inhibition of the LH and FSH responses to gonadotropin-releasing hormone occurs slowly. J Clin Endocrinol Metab.

1977. Jun;44(6):1142-53.
[12] Kerr JB, Sharpe RM. Follicle-stimulating hormone induction of Leydig cell maturation. Endocrinology. 1985 Jun;116(6):2592-604.
[13] Hartman ML, Crowe BJ, Biller BM, Ho KK, Clemmons DR, Chipman JJ; HyposCCS Advisory Board; U.S. HypoCCS Study Group. Which patients do not require a GH stimulation test for the diagnosis of adult GH deficiency? J Clin Endocrinol Metab. 2002 Feb;87(2):477-85.
[14] J Sex Med. 2011 Aug;8(8):2327-33. doi: 10.1111/j.1743-6109.2011.02354.x. Epub 2011 Jun 16. Hyperthyroidism: a risk factor for female sexual dysfunction. Atis G, Dalkilinc A, et al.
[15] Corona G, Wu FC,et al. Thyroid hormones and male sexual function. Int J Androl. 2012 Oct;35(5):668-79. doi: 10.1111/j.1365-2605.2012.01266.
[16] Fabrizio D'Ascenzo, Pierfrancesco Agostoni, et al. Atherosclerotic coronary plaque regression and the risk of adverse cardiovascular events: A meta-regression of randomized clinical trials Atherosclerosis, Volume: 226, Issue: 1, Pages: 178 to 185, Date: Monday, December 03, 2012.
[17] Abadilla KA, Dobs AS. Topical testosterone supplementation for the treatment of male hypogonadism. Drugs. 2012 Aug 20;72(12):1591-603. doi: 10.2165/11635620-000000000-00000.
[18] [Article in Spanish] Ruibal Francisco JL, Sánchez Burón P, et al. [Etiological, clinical and hormonal characteristics of a group of patients with permanent hypogonadism]. An Esp Pediatr. 1997 May;46(5):447-54.
[19] Davies JS, Hinds NP, Scanlon MF. Growth hormone deficiency and hypogonadism in a patient with multiple sclerosis. Clin Endocrinol (Oxf). 1996 Jan;44(1):117-9.
[20] Safarinejad MR. Evaluation of endocrine profile, hypothalamic-pituitary-testis axis and semen quality in multiple sclerosis. J Neuroendocrinol. 2008 Dec;20(12):1368-75. doi: 10.1111/j.1365-2826.2008.01791.
[21] Bates SL, Sharkey KA, et al. Vagal involvement in dietary regulation of nutrient transport. Am J Physiol. 1998 Mar;274(3 Pt 1):G552-60.
[22] Zhang XW, Liu ZH, et al. Androgen replacement therapy improves psychological distress and health-related quality of life in late onset hypogonadism patients in Chinese population. Chin Med J (Engl). 2012 Nov;125(21):3806-10.
[23] Aydogan U, Aydogdu A, et al. Increased frequency of anxiety, depression, quality of life and sexual life in young hypogonadotropic hypogonadal males and impacts of testosterone replacement therapy on these conditions. Endocr J. 2012 Dec 28;59(12):1099-105.
[24] Sher L, Grunebaum MF, et al. Testosterone levels in suicide attempters with

bipolar disorder. J Psychiatr Res. 2012 Oct;46(10):1267-71. doi: 10.1016/j.jpsychires.2012.06.016.

[25] Yaron M, Greenman Y, et al. Eff ect of testosterone replacement therapy on arterial stiffness in older hypogonadal men. Eur J Endocrinol. 2009 May;160(5):839-46. doi: 10.1530/EJE-09-0052.

[26] Albaaj F, Sivalingham M, et al. Prevalence of hypogonadism in male patients with renal failure. Postgrad Med J. 2006 Oct;82(972):693-6.

[27] Albaaj F, Sivalingham M, et al. Prevalence of hypogonadism in male patients with renal failure. Postgrad Med J. 2006 Oct;82(972):693-6.

[28] Accessed 22 March 2013 at http://www.usdoctor.com/testone.htm.

[29] Wagner AK, Brett CA, et al. Persistent hypogonadism influences estradiol synthesis, cognition and outcome in males after severe TBI. Brain Inj. 2012;26(10):1226-42. doi: 10.3109/02699052.2012.667594.

[30] Tanriverdi F, De Bellis A, et al. Five years prospective investigation of anterior pituitary function after traumatic brain injury: is hypopituitarism long-term after head trauma associated with autoimmunity? J Neurotrauma. 2013 Mar 7.

[31] Accessed online 22 March 2013. http://sports.espn.go.com/mlb/news/story?id=4148907.

[32] Accessed online 22 March 2013 at http://articles.latimes.com/2009/may/12/sports/sp-manny-dodgers12.

[33] Accessed online 22 March, 2013. http://online.wsj.com/article/SB124171191680796495.html.

[34] Rajender S, Monica MG, et al. Thyroid, spermatogenesis, and male infertility. Front Biosci (Elite Ed). 2011 Jun 1;3:843-55.

[35] D'Ascenzo F, Agostoni P, et al. Atherosclerotic coronary plaque regression and the risk of adverse cardiovascular events: a meta-regression of randomized clinical trials. Atherosclerosis. 2013 Jan;226(1):178-85. doi: 10.1016/j.atherosclerosis.2012.10.065.

[36] Rennert G, Rennert HS, et al. A case-control study of levothyroxine and the risk of colorectal cancer. J Natl Cancer Inst. 2010 Apr 21;102(8):568-72. doi: 10.1093/jnci/djq042.

[37] Bourre JM. Dietary omega-3 Fatty acids and psychiatry: mood, behaviour, stress, depression, dementia and aging. J Nutr Health Aging. 2005;9(1):31-8.

[38] Skulas-Ray AC, Kris-Etherton PM, et al. Dose-response effects of omega-3 fatty acids on triglycerides, inflammation, and endothelial function in healthy persons with moderate hypertriglyceridemia. Am J Clin Nutr. 2011 Feb;93(2):243-52. doi: 10.3945/ajcn.110.003871.

[39] Mo Q, Lu SF, Simon NG (April 2006). "Dehydroepiandrosterone and its metabolites: differential effects on androgen receptor trafficking and transcriptional activity". *J. Steroid Biochem. Mol. Biol.* **99**(1): 50–

8. doi:10.1016/j.jsbmb.2005.11.011. PMID 16524719.

[40] Thomas Scott (1996). *Concise Encyclopedia Biology*. Walter de Gruyter. p. 49. ISBN 978-3-11-010661-9. Retrieved 25 May 2012.

[41] Accessed 23 March, 2013 at http://www.lifeextensionvitamins.com/prcrhoforema.html.

[42] Safarinejad MR, Safarinejad S, et al. Effects of the reduced form of coenzyme Q10 (ubiquinol) on semen parameters in men with idiopathic infertility: a double-blind, placebo controlled, randomized study. J Urol. 2012 Aug;188(2):526-31. doi: 10.1016/j.juro.2012.03.131.

[43] Safarinejad MR. Efficacy of coenzyme Q10 on semen parameters, sperm function and reproductive hormones in infertile men. J Urol. 2009 Jul;182(1):237-48. doi: 10.1016/j.juro.2009.02.121.

[44] Kwiecinski GG, Petrie GI et al. Vitamin D is necessary for reproductive functions of the male rat. J Nutr. 1989 May;119(5):741-4.

[45] Benbrahim-Tallaa L, Tabone E, et al. Glutathione S-transferase alpha expressed in porcine Sertoli cells is under the control of follicle-stimulating hormone and testosterone. Biol Reprod. 2002 Jun;66(6):1734-42.

[46] Eichholzer M, Steinbrecher A, et al. Effects of selenium status, dietary glucosinolate intake and serum glutathione S-transferase α activity on the risk of benign prostatic hyperplasia. JU Int. 2012 Dec;110(11 Pt C):E879-85. doi: 10.1111/j.1464-410X.2012.11383.x.

[47] Erkkilä K, Hirvonen V, et al. N-acetyl-L-cysteine inhibits apoptosis in human male germ cells in vitro. J Clin Endocrinol Metab. 1998 Jul;83(7):2523-31.

[48] Fernandes GS, Gerardin DC, et al. Can vitamins C and E restore the androgen level and hypersensitivity of the vas deferens in hyperglycemic rats? Pharmacol Rep. 2011;63(4):983-91.

[49] O'Bryan MK, Schlatt S, et al. Inducible nitric oxide synthase in the rat testis: evidence for potential roles in both normal function and inflammation-mediated infertility. Biol Reprod. 2000 Nov;63(5):1285-93.

[50] Abd-Allah AR, Helal GK, et al. Pro-inflammatory and oxidative stress pathways which compromise sperm motility and survival may be altered by L-carnitine. Oxid Med Cell Longev. 2009 Apr-Jun;2(2):73-81.

[51]Accessed 22 March 2013 at http://www.ehow.com/how-does_5214641_amino-acid-l_ornithine-do_.html.

[52]Chausmer AB, Chavez C, et al. Calcitonin, zinc, and testicular function. Metabolism. 1989 Aug;38(8):714-7.

[53] Akinloye O, Arowojolu AO, et al. Selenium status of idiopathic infertile Nigerian males. Biol Trace Elem Res. 2005 Apr;104(1):9-18.

[54] Valentina VN, Marijan B, et al. Subclinical hypothyroidism and risk to carotid atherosclerosis. Arq Bras Endocrinol Metabol. 2011 Oct;55(7):475-80.

[55] Jiskra J, Límanová Z, et al. Autoimmune thyroid diseases in women with

157

breast cancer and colorectal cancer. Physiol Res. 2004;53(6):693-702.

[56] Hellevik AI, Asvold BO, et al. Thyroid function and cancer risk: a prospective population study. Cancer Epidemiol Biomarkers Prev. 2009 Feb;18(2):570-4. doi: 10.1158/1055-9965.EPI-08-0911.

[57] Rajender S, Monica MG, et al. Thyroid, spermatogenesis, and male infertility. Front Biosci (Elite Ed). 2011 Jun 1;3:843-55.

[58] Schachter M. Chemical, pharmacokinetic and pharmacodynamic properties of statins: an update. Fundam Clin Pharmacol. 2005 Feb;19(1):117-25.

[59] Lee K, Ahn TH, et al. The effects of statin and niacin on plaque stability, plaque regression, inflammation and oxidative stress in patients with mild to moderate coronary artery stenosis. Korean Circ J. 2011 Nov;41(11):641-8. doi: 10.4070/kcj.2011.41.11.641.

[60] Giltay EJ, Geleijnse JM, et al. No effects of n-3 fatty acid supplementation on serum total testosterone levels in older men: the Alpha Omega Trial. Int J Androl. 2012 Oct;35(5):680-7. doi: 10.1111/j.1365-2605.2012.01255.x.

[61] Ozcan ME, Banoglu R. Gonadal hormones in schizophrenia and mood disorders. Eur Arch Psychiatry Clin Neurosci. 2003 Aug;253(4):193-6.

[62] Xiaowei Z, Zhenhua L, et al. Testosterone therapy improves psychological distress and health-related quality of life in Chinese men with symptomatic late-onset hypogonadism patients. Aging Male. 2013 Jan 10.

[63] Ready RE, Friedman J, et al. Testosterone deficiency and apathy in Parkinson's disease: a pilot study. J Neurol Neurosurg Psychiatry. 2004 Sep;75(9):1323-6.

[64] Accessed 23 March 2013 at http://www.whitelotuseast.com/MultipleOrgasm.htm.

[65] Accessed 23 March 2013 at http://www.askmen.com/dating/love_tip_200/230_love_tip.html.

[66] Safarinejad MR. The effect of coenzyme Q_{10} supplementation on partner pregnancy rate in infertile men with idiopathic oligoasthenoteratozoospermia: an open-label prospective study. Int Urol Nephrol. 2012 Jun;44(3):689-700. doi: 10.1007/s11255-011-0081-0.

[67] Accessed 23 March 2013 at http://www.washingtonpost.com/blogs/blogpost/post/fenugreek-can-increase-male-libido/2011/06/20/AGOxpqcH_blog.html.

[68] Batirel HF, Naka Y, et al. Intravenous allicin improves pulmonary blood flow after ischemia-reperfusion injury in rats. J Cardiovasc Surg (Torino). 2002 Apr;43(2):175-9.

[69] Da Ros CT, Averbeck MA. Twenty-five milligrams of clomiphene citrate presents positive effect on treatment of male testosterone deficiency - a prospective study. Int Braz J Urol. 2012 Jul-Aug;38(4):512-8.

[70] Moskovic DJ, Katz DJ, Akhavan A, Park K, Mulhall JP. Clomiphene citrate is

safe and effective for long-term management of hypogonadism. BJU Int. 2012 Nov;110(10):1524-8. doi: 10.1111/j.1464-410X.2012.10968.x. Epub 2012 Mar 28.

[71] Kim ED, Crosnoe L, et al. The treatment of hypogonadism in men of reproductive age. Fertil Steril. 2012 Dec 6. pii: S0015-0282(12)02430-2. doi: 10.1016/j.fertnstert.2012.10.052.

[72] Shabsigh A, Kang Y, et al. Clomiphene citrate effects on testosterone/estrogen ratio in male hypogonadism. J Sex Med. 2005 Sep;2(5):716-21.

[73] Online at http://jeffreydach.com/2012/06/18/clomid-for-men-with-low-testosterone-by-jeffrey-dach-md.aspx. Accessed 14 Apr 2013.

[74] Online at http://www.allthingsmale.com/forum/archive/index.php/t-21073.html?s=5dabae4ca583ebda63123ebb00f8dda0. Accessed 14 Apr 2013.

[75] Liu Y, Li X. Molecular basis of cryptorchidism-induced infertility. Sci China Life Sci. 2010 Nov;53(11):1274-83. doi: 10.1007/s11427-010-4072-7.

[76] Lissner E. New nonhormonal contraceptive methods for men. Chang Men. 1992 Summer-Fall:24-5.

[77] Baazeem A, Belzile E, Ciampi A, et al. Varicocele and male factor infertility treatment: a new meta-analysis and review of the role of varicocele repair. Eur Urol. 2011 Oct;60(4):796-808. doi: 10.1016/j.eururo.2011.06.018.

[78] Mahmood, TA. Influences of Excess Adiposity on Reproductive Function. British Journal of Diabetes and Vascular Disease. 2009;9(5):197-199.

[79] Joo KJ, Kwon YW, Myung SC, Kim TH. The effects of smoking and alcohol intake on sperm quality: light and transmission electron microscopy findings. J Int Med Res. 2012;40(6):2327-35.

[80] Badawy ZS, Chohan KR, Whyte DA, et al. Cannabinoids inhibit the respiration of human sperm. Fertil Steril. 2009 Jun;91(6):2471-6. doi: 10.1016/j.fertnstert.2008.03.075.

[81] De Sanctis V, Ciccone S. Fertility preservation in adolescents with Klinefelter's syndrome. Pediatr Endocrinol Rev. 2010 Dec;8 Suppl 1:178-81.

[82] Ahmad A, Ahmed A, Patrizio P. Cystic fibrosis and fertility. Curr Opin Obstet Gynecol. 2013 Feb 19.

[83] Accessed 23 March 2013 at http://claircarecenter.com/ways-to-decode-omega-3-and-omegagize/

[84] Accessed 23 March 2013 at http://www.younglivinglink.com/?p=2521.

[85] Gurbuz C, Canat L, Atis G, et al. The role of serum testosterone to prostate-specific antigen ratio as a predictor of prostate cancer risk. Kaohsiung J Med Sci. 2012 Dec;28(12):649-53. doi: 10.1016/j.kjms.2012.01.003.

[86] Smith AM, Jones RD, Channer KS. The influence of sex hormones on pulmonary vascular reactivity: possible vasodilator therapies for the treatment of pulmonary hypertension. Curr Vasc Pharmacol. 2006 Jan;4(1):9-15.

[87] Golden SH, Maguire A, Ding J, Crouse JR, Cauley JA, Zacur H, Szklo M. Endogenous postmenopausal hormones and carotid atherosclerosis: a case-control study of the atherosclerosis risk in communities cohort. Am J Epidemiol. 2002 Mar 1;155(5):437-45.

[88] Dobrzycki S, Serwatka W, Nadlewski S, et al. An assessment of correlations between endogenous sex hormone levels and the extensiveness of coronary heart disease and the ejection fraction of the left ventricle in males. J Med Invest. 2003 Aug;50(3-4):162-9.

[89] Phillips GB, Pinkernell BH, Jing TY. Are major risk factors for myocardial infarction the major predictors of degree of coronary artery disease in men? Metabolism. 2004 Mar;53(3):324-9.

[90] Dzugan SA, Smith RA. Hypercholesterolemia treatment: a new hypothesis or just an accident? Med Hypothesis. 2002 Dec;59(6):751-6.

[91] Dzugan SA, Smith RA. Broad spectrum restoration in natural steroid hormones as possible treatment for hypercholesterolemia. Bull Urg Rec Med. 2002;3(2):278-84.

[92] English KM, Steeds R, Jones TH, Channer KS: Testosterone and coronary heart disease: is there a link? Q J Med 90:787–791, 1997.

[93] Anderson RA, Ludlam CA, Wu FC: Haemostatic effects of supraphysiological levels of testosterone in normal men. Thromb Haemost 74:693–697, 1995.

[94] Webb CM, McNeill JG, Hayward CS, Zeigler D, Collins P: Effects of testosterone on coronary vasomotor regulation in men with coronary heart disease. Circulation 100:1690–1696, 1999.

[95] Osuna JA, Gomez-Perez R, Arata-Bellabarba G, Villaroel V. Relationship between BMI, total testosterone, sex hormone-binding-globulin, leptin, insulin and insulin resistance in obese men. Arch Androl. 2006 Sep-Oct;52(5):355-61.

[96] Simon D, Charles MA, Nahoul K, Orssaud G, Kremski J, Hully V, Joubert E, Papoz L, Eschwege E: Association between plasma total testosterone and cardiovascular risk factors in healthy adult men: the Telecom Study. J Clin Endocrinol Metab 82:682–685, 1997.

[97] Abrams D. Use of androgens in patients who have HIV/AIDS: what we know about the effect of androgens on wasting and lipodystrophy. AIDS Read. 2001 Mar;11(3):149-56.

[98] Osuna JA, Gomez-Perez R, Arata-Bellabarba G, Villaroel V. Relationship between BMI, total testosterone, sex hormone-binding-globulin, leptin, insulin and insulin resistance in obese men. Arch Androl. 2006 Sep-Oct;52(5):355-61.

[99] Hogervorst E, Bandelow S, Combrinck M, Smith AD. Low free testosterone is an independent risk factor for Alzheimer's disease. Exp Gerontol. 2004 Nov-Dec;39(11-12):1633-9.

[100] Winters, SJ. Current Status of Testosterone Replacement Therapy in Men.

Arch Fam Med. 1999;8:257-263.

[101] Carrier S, Zvara P, Lue TF. Erectile dysfunction. *Endocrinol Metab Clin North Am.* 1994;23:773-782.

[102] Shifren JL, Braunstein GD, Simon JA, Casson PR, Buster JE, Redmond GP, Burki RE, Ginsburg ES, Rosen RC, Leiblum SR, Caramelli KE, Mazer NA. Transdermal testosterone treatment in women with impaired sexual function after oophorectomy. N Engl J Med. 2000 Sep 7;343(10):682-8.

[103] Mooradian AD, Morley JE, Korenman SG. Biological actions of androgens. *Endocr Rev.* 1987;8:1-28.

[104] Veldhuis JD, Keenan DM, Mielke K, Miles JM, Bowers CY. Testosterone supplementation in healthy older men drives GH and IGF-I secretion without potentiating peptidyl secretagogue efficacy. Eur J Endocrinol. 2005 Oct;153(4):577-86.

[105] Yael Waknine. Testosterone Replacement Improves Exercise Capacity in Men With CHF. [online] Available on Medscape Medical News 2005. © 2005 Medscape at www.medscape.com/viewarticle/506223

[106] Malkin CJ, Pugh PJ, West JN, van Beek EJ, Jones TH, Channer KS. Testosterone therapy in men with moderate severity heart failure: a double-blind randomized placebo controlled trial. Eur Heart J. 2006 Jan;27(1):57-64.

[107] Walston, J; Hadley, EC; Ferrucci, L; Guralnik, JM; Newman, AB; Studenski, SA; Ershler, WB; Harris, T; Fried, LP. Research Agenda for Frailty in Older Adults. J Am Geriatr Soc. 2006;54(6):991-1001. ©2006 Blackwell Publishing.

[108] Hackney AC, Moore AW, Brownlee KK. Testosterone and endurance exercise: development of the "exercise-hypogonadal male condition". Acta Physiol Hung. 2005;92(2):121-37.

[109] Demling RH. The role of anabolic hormones for wound healing in catabolic States. J Burns Wounds. 2005 Jan 17;4:e2.

[110] Hardman MJ, Ashcroft GS. Hormonal influences on wound healing: a review of current experimental data. WOUNDS. 2005;17(11):313-320.

[111] Muller M; Aleman A; Grobbee DE; de Haan EH; van der Schouw YT. Endogenous sex hormone levels and cognitive function in aging men: is there an optimal level? Neurology. 2005; 64(5):866-71 (ISSN: 1526-632X).

[112] Brian C. Lund, Pharm.D., Kristine A. Bever-Stille, Pharm.D., and Paul J. Perry, Ph.D. Testosterone and Andropause: The Feasibility of Testosterone Replacement Therapy in Elderly Men. Pharmacotherapy 19(8):951-956, 1999. © 1999 Pharmacotherapy Publications.

[113] American College of Endocrinologists and American Association of Clinical Endocrinologists. *Guidelines for the Evaluation and Treatment of Male Sexual Dysfunction.* American College of Endocrinologists and American Association of Clinical Endocrinologists; 1998:4.

[114] Aversa A, Isidori AM, De Martino MU, et al. Androgens and penile erection

evidence for a direct relationship between free testosterone and cavernous vasodilation in men with ED. Clin Endocrinol (Oxf). 2000;53:517-522.

[115] [Article in Chinese] Chen X, Li X, Huang HY, Li X, Lin JF. [Effects of testosterone on insulin receptor substrate-1 and glucose transporter 4 expression in cells sensitive to insulin] Zhonghua Yi Xue Za Zhi. 2006 Jun 6;86(21):1474-7.

[116] Braga-Basaria M, Dobs AS, Muller DC, Carducci MA, John M, Egan J, Basaria S. Metabolic syndrome in men with prostate cancer undergoing long-term androgen-deprivation therapy. J Clin Oncol. 2006 Aug 20;24(24):3979-83.

[117] Svartberg J. Epidemiology: testosterone and the metabolic syndrome. Int J Impot Res. 2006 Jul 20.

[118] Fogari R, Preti P, Zoppi A, Fogari E, Rinaldi A, Corradi L, Mugellini A. Serum testosterone levels and arterial blood pressure in the elderly. Hypertens Res. 2005 Aug;28(8):625-30.

[119] Huisman HW, Schutte AE, Van Rooyen JM, Malan NT, Malan L, Schutte R, Kruger A. The influence of testosterone on blood pressure and risk factors for cardiovascular disease in a black South African population. Ethn Dis. 2006 Summer;16(3):693-8.

[120] Vondracek, SF; Hansen, LB. Current Approaches to the Management of Osteoporosis in Men. Am J Health-Syst Pharm 61(17):1801-1811, 2004. © 2004 American Society of Health-System Pharmacists.

[121] Isidori AM, Giannetta E, Greco EA, Gianfrilli D, Bonifacio V, Isidori A, Lenzi A, Fabbri A. Effects of testosterone on body composition, bone metabolism and serum lipid profile in middle-aged men: a meta-analysis. Clin Endocrinol (Oxf). 2005 Sep;63(3):280-93.

[122] Reported by By Karla Gale. Testosterone May Slow Progress of MS in Men. Reuters Health Information 2006. © 2006 Reuters Ltd. [online] Available on Medscape® at www.medscape.com/viewarticle/529199.

[123] Markianos M; Panas M; Kalfakis N; Vassilopoulos D. Plasma testosterone in male patients with Huntington's disease: relations to severity of illness and dementia. Ann Neurol. 2005; 57(4):520-5 (ISSN: 0364-5134).

[124] Moffat SD. Effects of testosterone on cognitive and brain aging in elderly men. Ann N Y Acad Sci. 2005; 1055:80-92 (ISSN: 0077-8923).

[125] Bialek M, Zaremba P, Borowicz KK, Czuczwar SJ. Neuroprotective role of testosterone in the nervous system. Pol J Pharmacol. 2004 Sep-Oct;56(5):509-18.

[126] Finazzi G, Gregg XT, Barbui T, Prchal JT. Idiopathic erythrocytosis and other non-clonal polycythemias. Best Pract Res Clin Haematol. 2006;19(3):471-82.

[127] Ferrucci L, Maggio M, Bandinelli S, Basaria S, Lauretani F, Ble A, Valenti G, Ershler WB, Guralnik JM, Longo DL. Low testosterone levels and the risk of

anemia in older men and women. Arch Intern Med. 2006 Jul 10;166(13):1380-8.

[128] McVary KT; McKenna KE. The relationship between erectile dysfunction and lower urinary tract symptoms: epidemiological, clinical, and basic science evidence. Curr Urol Rep. 2004; 5(4):251-7 (ISSN: 1527-2737).

[129] Kaminetsky J. Comorbid LUTS and erectile dysfunction: optimizing their management. Curr Med Res Opin. 2006 Dec;22(12):2497-506.

[130] Spector TD, Perry LA, Tubb G, Silman AJ, Huskisson EC. Low free testosterone levels in rheumatoid arthritis. Ann Rheum Dis. 1988 Jan;47(1):65-8.

[131] Cutolo M, Balleari E, Giusti M, Monachesi M, Accardo S. Sex hormone status of male patients with rheumatoid arthritis: evidence of low serum concentrations of testosterone at baseline and after human chorionic gonadotropin stimulation. Arthritis Rheum. 1988 Oct;31(10):1314-7.

[132] Rhoden EL; Morgentaler A. Testosterone replacement therapy in hypogonadal men at high risk for prostate cancer: results of 1 year of treatment in men with prostatic intraepithelial neoplasia. J Urol. 2003; 170(6 Pt 1):2348-51 (ISSN: 0022-5347)

[133] Smith AM, English KM, Malkin CJ, Jones RD, Jones TH, Channer KS. Testosterone does not adversely affect fibrinogen or tissue plasminogen activator (tPA) and plasminogen activator inhibitor-1 (PAI-1) levels in 46 men with chronic stable angina. Eur J Endocrinol. 2005 Feb;152(2):285-91.

[134] Orwoll E, Lambert LC, Marshall LM, Blank J, Barrett-Connor E, Cauley J, Ensrud K, Cummings SR; Osteoporotic Fractures in Men Study Group. Endogenous testosterone levels, physical performance, and fall risk in older men. Arch Intern Med. 2006 Oct 23;166(19):2124-31.

[135] Gurbuz C, Canat L, Atis G, et al. The role of serum testosterone to prostate-specific antigen ratio as a predictor of prostate cancer risk. Kaohsiung J Med Sci. 2012 Dec;28(12):649-53. doi: 10.1016/j.kjms.2012.01.003.

[136] Pastuszak AW, Pearlman AM, Lai WS, et al. Testosterone Replacement Therapy in Patients with Prostate Cancer After Radical Prostatectomy. J Urol. 2013 Feb 7. pii: S0022-5347(13)00259-0. doi: 10.1016/j.juro.2013.02.002.

[137] Morgentaler A. Testosterone therapy in men with prostate cancer: scientific and ethical considerations. J Urol. 2013 Jan;189(1 Suppl):S26-33. doi: 10.1016/j.juro.2012.11.028.

[138] No author listed (2007) Testicular Cancer. [Online] University of Miami Leonard M. Miller School of Medicine Publishing. Available from: http://urology.med.miami.edu/x44.xml [Accessed 15th Jan 2013].

[139] Soisson V, Brailly-Tabard S, Empana JP, et al. Low plasma testosterone and elevated carotid intima-media thickness: importance of low-grade inflammation in elderly men. Atherosclerosis. 2012 Jul;223(1):244-9. doi: 10.1016/j.atherosclerosis.2012.05.009.

[140] Vlachopoulos C, Ioakeimidis N, Terentes-Printzios D, et al. Plasma total testosterone and incident cardiovascular events in hypertensive patients. Am J Hypertens. 2013 Mar;26(3):373-81. doi: 10.1093/ajh/hps056.

[141] Garcia-Cruz E, Piqueras M, Huguet J, et al. Hypertension, dyslipidemia and overweight are related to lower testosterone levels in a cohort of men undergoing prostate biopsy. Int J Impot Res. 2012 May-Jun;24(3):110-3. doi: 10.1038/ijir.2011.55.

[142] Garcia-Cruz E, Piqueras M, Huguet J, et al. Hypertension, dyslipidemia and overweight are related to lower testosterone levels in a cohort of men undergoing prostate biopsy. Int J Impot Res. 2012 May-Jun;24(3):110-3. doi: 10.1038/ijir.2011.55.

[143] Pastuszak AW, Badhiwala N, Lipshultz LI, et al. Depression is correlated with the psychological and physical aspects of sexual dysfunction in men. Int J Impot Res. 2013 Mar 7. doi: 10.1038/ijir.2013.4.

[144] Lee K, Ahn TH, Kang WC, Han SH, et al. The effects of statin and niacin on plaque stability, plaque regression, inflammation and oxidative stress in patients with mild to moderate coronary artery stenosis. Korean Circ J. 2011 Nov;41(11):641-8. doi: 10.4070/kcj.2011.41.11.641.

[145] Gottlieb I, Agarwal S, Gautam S, et al. Aortic plaque regression as determined by magnetic resonance imaging with high-dose and low-dose statin therapy. J Cardiovasc Med (Hagerstown). 2008 Jul;9(7):700-6. doi: 10.2459/JCM.0b013e3282f447c3.

[146] Nohara R, Daida H, Hata M, et al. Effect of Long-Term Intensive Lipid-Lowering Therapy With Rosuvastatin on Progression of Carotid Intima-Media Thickness. Circ J. 2013 Mar 14.

[147] Takamura N, Akilzhanova A, Hayashida N, et al. Thyroid function is associated with carotid intima-media thickness in euthyroid subjects. Atherosclerosis. 2009 Jun;204(2):e77-81. doi: 10.1016/j.atherosclerosis.2008.09.022.

[148] Yang HB, Zhao XY, Zhang JY, et al. Pioglitazone induces regression and stabilization of coronary atherosclerotic plaques in patients with impaired glucose tolerance. Diabet Med. 2012 Mar;29(3):359-65. doi: 10.1111/j.1464-5491.2011.03458.x.

[149] Ferwana M, Firwana B, Hasan R, et al. Pioglitazone and risk of bladder cancer: a meta-analysis of controlled studies. Diabet Med. 2013 Jan 28. doi: 10.1111/dme.12144.

[150] von der Thüsen JH, Borensztajn KS, et al. IGF-1 has plaque-stabilizing effects in atherosclerosis by altering vascular smooth muscle cell phenotype. Am J Pathol. 2011 Feb;178(2):924-34. doi: 10.1016/j.ajpath.2010.10.007.

[151] Chhatriwalla AK, Nicholls SJ, et al. Low levels of low-density lipoprotein cholesterol and blood pressure and progression of coronary atherosclerosis. J

Am Coll Cardiol. 2009 Mar 31;53(13):1110-5. doi: 10.1016/j.jacc.2008.09.065.

[152] Romiti A, Martelletti P, at al. Low plasma testosterone levels in cluster headache. Cephalalgia. 1983 Mar;3(1):41-4.

[153] Saad F. Androgen therapy in men with testosterone deficiency: can testosterone reduce the risk of cardiovascular disease? Diabetes Metab Res Rev. 2012 Dec;28 Suppl 2:52-9. doi: 10.1002/dmrr.2354.

[154] Silberstein S, Newman L, et al. Efficacy Endpoints in Migraine Clinical Trials: The Importance of Assessing Freedom from Pain. Curr Med Res Opin. 2013 Mar 20.

[155] Soisson V, Brailly-Tabard S, Empana JP, et al. Low plasma testosterone and elevated carotid intima-media thickness: importance of low-grade inflammation in elderly men. Atherosclerosis. 2012 Jul;223(1):244-9. doi: 10.1016/j.atherosclerosis.2012.05.009.

[156] Dockery F, Bulpitt CJ, Donaldson M, Fernandez S, Rajkumar C. The relationship between androgens and arterial stiffness in older men. J Am Geriatr Soc. 2003 Nov;51(11):1627-32.

[157] Rosmond R, Wallerius S, Wanger P, Martin L, Holm G, Bjorntorp P. A 5-year follow-up study of disease incidence in men with an abnormal hormone pattern. J Intern Med. 2003 Oct;254(4):386-90.

[158] Cohen PG. Aromatase, adiposity, aging and disease. The hypogonadal-metabolic-atherogenic-disease and aging connection. Med Hypotheses. 2001 Jun;56(6):702-8.

[159] Sun MY, Chen TC, Lee YL. Hypothyroidism and cerebral infarction: a case report and literature review. Acta Neurol Taiwan. 2006 Sep;15(3):197-200.

[160] Squizzato A, Gerdes VE, Brandjes DP, Buller HR, Stam J. Thyroid diseases and cerebrovascular disease. Stroke. 2005 Oct;36(10):2302-10.

[161] Ridker PM; Cook NR; Lee IM; Gordon D; Gaziano JM; Manson JE; Hennekens CH; Buring JE. A randomized trial of low-dose aspirin in the primary prevention of cardiovascular disease in women. N Engl J Med. 2005; 352(13):1293-304 (ISSN: 1533-4406).

[162] Pinto A, Di Raimondo D, Tuttolomondo A, Fernandez P, Arna V, Licata G. Twenty-four hour ambulatory blood pressure monitoring to evaluate effects on blood pressure of physical activity in hypertensive patients. Clin J Sport Med. 2006 May;16(3):238-43.

[163] Oczkowski W. Complexity of the relation between physical activity and stroke: a meta-analysis. Clin J Sport Med. 2005; 15(5):399 (ISSN: 1050-642X).

[164] Alevizos, A; Lentzas, J; Kokkoris, S; Mariolis, A; Korantzopoulos, P. Physical Activity and Stroke Risk. Int J Clin Pract 59(8):922-930, 2005. © 2005 Blackwell Publishing.

[165] Chobanian AV, Bakris GL, Black HR, et al. The Seventh Report of the Joint

National Committee on Prevention, Detection, Evaluation, and Treatment of High Blood Pressure: the JNC 7 report. JAMA. 2003;289:2560-2572.

[166] Wexler R, Aukerman G. Nonpharmacologic strategies for managing hypertension. Am Fam Physician. 2006 Jun 1;73(11):1953-6.

[167] Svetkey, LP; Simons-Morton, DG; Proschan, MA; Sacks, FM; Conlin, PR; Harsha, D; Moore, TJ; for the DASH-Sodium Collaborative Research Group. Effect of the Dietary Approaches to Stop Hypertension Diet and Reduced Sodium Intake on Blood Pressure Control. J Clin Hypertens 6(7):373-381, 2004. © 2004 Le Jacq Communications, Inc.

[168] US Department of Health and Human Services. JNC 7 Express. The Seventh Report of the Joint National Committee on Prevention, Detection, Evaluation, and Treatment of High Blood Pressure. Available on the NHLBI Web site at http://www.nhlbi.nih.gov or from the NHLBI Health Information Center, PO Box 30105, Bethesda, MD 20824-0105. Phone 301-592-8573 or 240-629-3255 (TTY); Fax: 301-592-8563.

[169] Major Outcomes in High-Risk Hypertensive Patients Randomized to Angiotensin-Converting Enzyme Inhibitor or Calcium Channel Blocker vs Diuretic: The Antihypertensive and Lipid-Lowering Treatment to Prevent Heart Attack Trial (ALLHAT). The ALLHAT Officers and Coordinators for the ALLHAT Collaborative Research Group. JAMA. 2002;288:2981-3007.

[170] Wannamethee SG ; Shaper AG ; Walker M. Overweight and obesity and weight change in middle aged men: impact on cardiovascular disease and diabetes. J Epidemiol Community Health. 2005; 59(2):134-9 (ISSN: 0143-005X).

[171] Wannamethee SG ; Shaper AG ; Walker M. Overweight and obesity and weight change in middle aged men: impact on cardiovascular disease and diabetes. J Epidemiol Community Health. 2005; 59(2):134-9 (ISSN: 0143-005X).

[172] Carlson LA. Niaspan, the prolonged release preparation of nicotinic acid (niacin), the broad-spectrum lipid drug. Int J Clin Pract. 2004; 58(7):706-13 (ISSN: 1368-5031).

[173] Edwards, L.E. Ask the Experts about Cardiology for Advanced Practice Nurses - From Medscape Nurses. What Should I Know About Niacin Preparations and Dyslipidemia? [online] Available at www.medscape.com/viewarticle/501893. Accessed 2006 13 July.

[174] Carlson LA. Niaspan, the prolonged release preparation of nicotinic acid (niacin), the broad-spectrum lipid drug. Int J Clin Pract. 2004; 58(7):706-13 (ISSN: 1368-5031).

[175] Capuzzi, DM; Morgan, JM; Carey, CM; Intenzo, C; Tulenko, T; Kearney, D; Walker, K; Cressman, MD. Rosuvastatin Alone or With Extended-Release Niacin: A New Therapeutic Option for Patients With Combined Hyperlipidemia.

Prev Cardiol 7(4):176-181, 2004. © 2004 Le Jacq Communications, Inc.

[176] Oger E, Lacut K, Le Gal G, Couturaud F, Guenet D, Abalain JH, Roguedas AM, Mottier D; EDITH COLLABORATIVE STUDY GROUP. Hyperhomocysteinemia and low B vitamin levels are independently associated with venous thromboembolism: results from the EDITH study: a hospital-based case-control study. J Thromb Haemost. 2006 Apr;4(4):793-9.

[177] Flicker L, Vasikaran SD, Thomas J, Acres JM, Norman P, Jamrozik K, Hankey GJ, Almeida OP. Efficacy of B vitamins in lowering homocysteine in older men: maximal effects for those with B12 deficiency and hyperhomocysteinemia. Stroke. 2006 Feb;37(2):547-9. Epub 2005 Dec 22.

[178] Yaggi, H.K. Obstructive Sleep Apnea as a Risk Factor for Stroke and Death. The New England Journal of Medicine, Nov. 10, 2005; vol 353: pp 2034-2041.

[179] Shivalkar B, Van de Heyning C, Kerremans M, Rinkevich D, Verbraecken J, De Backer W, Vrints C. Obstructive sleep apnea syndrome: more insights on structural and functional cardiac alterations, and the effects of treatment with continuous positive airway pressure. J Am Coll Cardiol. 2006 Apr 4;47(7):1433-9.

[180] Kostis JB, Rosen RC, Wilson AC. Central nervous system effects of HMG CoA reductase inhibitors: lovastatin and pravastatin on sleep and cognitive performance in patients with hypercholesterolemia. J Clin Pharmacol. 1994 Oct;34(10):989-96.

[181] Mega JL, Morrow DA, Cannon CP, Murphy S, Cairns R, Ridker PM, Braunwald E. Cholesterol, C-reactive protein, and cerebrovascular events following intensive and moderate statin therapy. J Thromb Thrombolysis. 2006 Aug;22(1):71-6.

[182] Hong H, Zeng JS, Kreulen DL, Kaufman DI, Chen AF. Atorvastatin Protects Against Cerebral Infarction via Inhibiting NADPH Oxidase-Derived Superoxide in Ischemic Stroke. Am J Physiol Heart Circ Physiol. 2006 Jun 9.

[183] Genser B, Marz W. Low density lipoprotein cholesterol, statins and cardiovascular events: a meta-analysis. Clin Res Cardiol. 2006 Jun 20.

[184] Amarenco P, Labreuche J, Lavallee P, Touboul PJ. Stroke. 2004 Dec;35(12):2902-9. Statins in stroke prevention and carotid atherosclerosis: systematic review and up-to-date meta-analysis.

[185] The Stroke Prevention by Aggressive Reduction in Cholesterol Levels (SPARCL) Investigators. High-dose atorvastatin after stroke or transient ischemic attack. N Engl J Med. 2006;355:459-559.

[186] Chan KY ; Boucher ES ; Gandhi PJ ; Silva MA. HMG-CoA reductase inhibitors for lowering elevated levels of C-reactive protein. Am J Health Syst Pharm. 2004; 61(16):1676-81 (ISSN: 1079-2082).

[187] McCarey DW, McInnes IB, Madhok R, et al. Trial of atorvastatin in rheumatoid arthritis (TARA): a double-blind, randomized placebo-controlled

trial. *Lancet* 2004; 363:2015-2021.

[188] Verma A, Ranganna KM, Reddy RS, Verma M, Gordon NF. Effect of rosuvastatin on C-reactive protein and renal function in patients with chronic kidney disease. Am J Cardiol. 2005 Nov 1;96(9):1290-2. Epub 2005 Sep 8.

[189] Sironi L, Gianazza E, Gelosa P, Guerrini U, Nobili E, Gianella A, Cremonesi B, Paoletti R, Tremoli E. Rosuvastatin, but not simvastatin, provides end-organ protection in stroke-prone rats by antiinflammatory effects. Arterioscler Thromb Vasc Biol. 2005 Mar;25(3):598-603. Epub 2005 Jan 27.

[190] Bouzan C, Cohen JT, Connor WE, Kris-Etherton PM, Gray GM, Konig A, Lawrence RS, Savitz DA, Teutsch SM. A quantitative analysis of fish consumption and stroke risk. Am J Prev Med. 2005 Nov;29(4):347-52.

[191] Iso H; Rexrode KM; Stampfer MJ; Manson JE; Colditz GA; Speizer FE; Hennekens CH; Willett WC. Intake of fish and omega-3 fatty acids and risk of stroke in women. JAMA. 2001; 285(3):304-12 (ISSN: 0098-7484).

[192] Tomer A, Kasey S, Connor WE, Clark S, Harker LA, Eckman JR. Reduction of pain episodes and prothrombotic activity in sickle cell disease by dietary n-3 fatty acids. Thromb Haemost. 2001 Jun;85(6):966-74.

[193] Singer DE, Albers GW, Dalen JE, Go AS, Halperin JL, Manning WJ. Antithrombotic therapy in atrial fibrillation: the Seventh ACCP Conference on Antithrombotic and Thrombolytic Therapy. Chest. 2004 Sep;126(3 Suppl):429S-456S.

[194] Singer DE, Albers GW, Dalen JE, Go AS, Halperin JL, Manning WJ. Antithrombotic therapy in atrial fibrillation: the Seventh ACCP Conference on Antithrombotic and Thrombolytic Therapy. Chest. 2004 Sep;126(3 Suppl):429S-456S.

[195] Singer DE, Albers GW, Dalen JE, Go AS, Halperin JL, Manning WJ. Antithrombotic therapy in atrial fibrillation: the Seventh ACCP Conference on Antithrombotic and Thrombolytic Therapy. Chest. 2004 Sep;126(3 Suppl):429S-456S.

[196] Singer DE, Albers GW, Dalen JE, Go AS, Halperin JL, Manning WJ. Antithrombotic therapy in atrial fibrillation: the Seventh ACCP Conference on Antithrombotic and Thrombolytic Therapy. Chest. 2004 Sep;126(3 Suppl):429S-456S.

[197] Wellington K. Rosiglitazone/Metformin. Drugs. 2005; 65(11):1581-92; discussion 1593-4 (ISSN: 0012-6667)

[198] Wellington K. Rosiglitazone/Metformin. Drugs. 2005; 65(11):1581-92; discussion 1593-4 (ISSN: 0012-6667)

[199] Ferrannini E, Dormandy J. Results of PROactive. Program and abstracts of the European Association for the Study of Diabetes 41st Annual Meeting; September 12-15, 2005; Athens, Greece.

[200] Ferrannini E, Dormandy J. Results of PROactive. Program and abstracts of

the European Association for the Study of Diabetes 41st Annual Meeting; September 12-15, 2005; Athens, Greece.

[201] Samaha FF, Szapary PO, et al. Effects of rosiglitazone on lipids, adipokines, and inflammatory markers in nondiabetic patients with low high-density lipoprotein cholesterol and metabolic syndrome. Arterioscler Thromb Vasc Biol. 2006 Mar;26(3):624-30. Epub 2005 Dec 15.

[202] Hussein Z, Wentworth JM, et al.Effectiveness and side effects of thiazolidinediones for type 2 diabetes: real-life experience from a tertiary hospital. Med J Aust. 2004 Nov 15;181(10):536-9.

[203] Ferrannini E, Dormandy J. Results of PROactive. Program and abstracts of the European Association for the Study of Diabetes 41st Annual Meeting; September 12-15, 2005; Athens, Greece.

[204] The DREAM (Diabetes Reduction Assessment with ramipril and rosiglitazone Medication) Trial Investigators. Effect of rosiglitazone on the frequency of diabetes in patients with impaired glucose tolerance or impaired fasting glucose: a randomized controlled trial. The Lancet. Published Online September 15, 2006. DOI:10.1016/S0140-6736(06)69420-8.

[205] Koshiyama H, Shimono D, Kuwamura N, Minamikawa J, Nakamura Y. Inhibitory effect of pioglitazone on carotid arterial wall thickness in type 2 diabetes. J Clin Endocrinol Metab. 2001;86:3452-3456.

[206] Brunetti P. Will the treatment of insulin resistance reduce cardiovascular disease? Program and abstracts of the 37th Annual Meeting of the European Association for the Study of Diabetes (EASD); September 9-13, 2001; Glasgow, United Kingdom. Symposium.

[207] Brunetti P. Will the treatment of insulin resistance reduce cardiovascular disease? Program and abstracts of the 37th Annual Meeting of the European Association for the Study of Diabetes (EASD); September 9-13, 2001; Glasgow, United Kingdom. Symposium.

[208] Brunetti P. Will the treatment of insulin resistance reduce cardiovascular disease? Program and abstracts of the 37th Annual Meeting of the European Association for the Study of Diabetes (EASD); September 9-13, 2001; Glasgow, United Kingdom. Symposium.

[209] Ferrannini E, Dormandy J. Results of PROactive. Program and abstracts of the European Association for the Study of Diabetes 41st Annual Meeting; September 12-15, 2005; Athens, Greece.

[210] Ferrannini E, Dormandy J. Results of PROactive. Program and abstracts of the European Association for the Study of Diabetes 41st Annual Meeting; September 12-15, 2005; Athens, Greece.

[211] Ferrannini E, Dormandy J. Results of PROactive. Program and abstracts of the European Association for the Study of Diabetes 41st Annual Meeting; September 12-15, 2005; Athens, Greece.

[212] Ferrannini E, Dormandy J. Results of PROactive. Program and abstracts of the European Association for the Study of Diabetes 41st Annual Meeting; September 12-15, 2005; Athens, Greece.

[213] Chu CS, Lee KT, Lee MY, Su HM, Voon WC, Sheu SH, Lai WT. Effects of rosiglitazone alone and in combination with atorvastatin on nontraditional markers of cardiovascular disease in patients with type 2 diabetes mellitus. Am J Cardiol. 2006 Mar 1;97(5):646-50.

[214] Shinohara K, Shoiji T, Emoto M, et al. Insulin resistance as an independent predictor of cardiovascular mortality in patients with end-stage renal disease. J Am Soc Nephrol 2002;13: 1894-900.

[215] Stocker DJ, Taylor AJ, Langley RW, Jezior MR, Vigersky RA. A randomized trial of the effects of rosiglitazone and metformin on inflammation and subclinical atherosclerosis in patients with type 2 diabetes. Am Heart J. 2007 Mar;153(3):445.e1-6.

[216] Mensink M, Hesselink MK, Russell AP, Schaart G, Sels JP, Schrauwen P. Improved skeletal muscle oxidative enzyme activity and restoration of PGC-1alpha and PPARbeta/delta gene expression upon rosiglitazone treatment in obese patients with type 2 diabetes mellitus. Int J Obes (Lond). 2007 Feb 20.

[217] Tahan V, Eren F, Avsar E, Yavuz D, Yuksel M, Emekli E, Imeryuz N, Celikel C, Uzun H, Haklar G, Tozun N. Rosiglitazone Attenuates Liver Inflammation in a Rat Model of Nonalcoholic Steatohepatitis. Dig Dis Sci. 2007 Apr 10.

[218] Berhanu P, Kipnes MS, Khan MA, Perez AT, Kupfer SF, Spanheimer RC, Demissie S, Fleck PR. Effects of pioglitazone on lipid and lipoprotein profiles in patients with type 2 diabetes and dyslipidaemia after treatment conversion from rosiglitazone while continuing stable statin therapy. Diab Vasc Dis Res. 2006 May;3(1):39-44.

[219] Haberbosch W. [Effects of thiazolidinediones on dyslipidemia in patients with type 2 diabetes. Are all equally vasoprotective?] [Article in German] Herz. 2007 Feb;32(1):51-7.

[220] [no author listed] Clot busting drugs for stroke: advantages for patients - and U.S. health care costs. (Mayo Clinic physician studies potential savings by increasing use of drug for stroke victims.). Mayo Clinic News. Mayo Clinic in Arizona. Tuesday, October 18, 2005. [online] Available at www.mayoclinic.org/news2005-sct/3076.html.

[221] Sicotte NL, Giesser BS, Tandon V, et al. Testosterone treatment in multiple sclerosis: a pilot study. Arch Neurol. 2007 May;64(5):683-8.

[222] Spence RD, Voskuhl RR. Neuroprotective effects of estrogens and androgens in CNS inflammation and neurodegeneration. Front Neuroendocrinol. 2012 Jan;33(1):105-15. doi: 10.1016/j.yfrne.2011.12.001.

[223] Bondanelli M, De Marinis L, Ambrosio MR, et al. Occurrence of pituitary

dysfunction following traumatic brain injury. J Neurotrauma. 2004 Jun;21(6):685-96.

[224] Seidman SN. Testosterone deficiency and mood in aging men: pathogenic and therapeutic interactions. World J Biol Psychiatry. 2003 Jan;4(1):14-20.

[225] Wilkinson CW, Pagulayan KF, Petrie EC, et al. High prevalence of chronic pituitary and target-organ hormone abnormalities after blast-related mild traumatic brain injury. Front Neurol. 2012;3:11. doi: 10.3389/fneur.2012.00011.

[226] [No authors listed] Contraceptive efficacy of testosterone-induced azoospermia in normal men. World Health Organization Task Force on methods for the regulation of male fertility. Lancet. 1990 Oct 20;336(8721):955-9.

[227] Purser, DC, MD; Radley, K. Program120: A Physician's Textbook of Preventive Medicine. Lindon. Aesthetica Preventive Medicine Institute Publishing, 2007.

[228] Jackson G, Boon N, Eardley I, et al. Erectile dysfunction and coronary artery disease prediction: evidence-based guidance and consensus. Int J Clin Pract. 2010 Jun;64(7):848-57. doi: 10.1111/j.1742-1241.2010.02410.x.

[229] Nichols WW, O'Rourke MF. McDonald's Blood Flow in Arteries. London, United Kingdom: Arnold; 2005.

[230] Mitka M. 1998 NObel Prize winners are announced: three discoverers of nitric oxide activity. JAMA. 1998 Nov 18;280(19):1648.

[231] Dockery F, Bulpitt CJ, et al. Effect of androgen suppression compared with androgen receptor blockade on arterial stiffness in men with prostate cancer. J Androl. 2009 Jul-Aug;30(4):410-5. doi: 10.2164/jandrol.108.006924. Epub 2009 Jan 22.

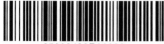

Made in the USA
Lexington, KY
30 March 2019